DR DAVID HASLAM

BULIMIA

A Guide for Sufferers
and their Families

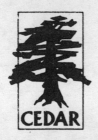

CEDAR

A Mandarin Paperback
BULIMIA

First published in Great Britain 1994
as a Cedar Original
by Mandarin Paperbacks
an imprint of Reed Consumer Books Ltd
Michelin House, 81 Fulham Road, London SW3 6RB
and Auckland, Melbourne, Singapore and Toronto

Reprinted 1994

Copyright © Dr David Haslam 1994
The author has asserted his moral rights

A CIP catalogue record for this title
is available from the British Library
ISBN 0 7493 1658 6

Printed and bound in Great Britain
by Cox & Wyman Ltd, Reading, Berks

Bulimia

A Guide for Sufferers and their Families

Dr David Haslam is a freelance
journalist and practising family
doctor. He is the author of *The
Mothercare Guide For The Expectant
Father*, *Travelling With Children*,
Parent Stress, *Eat It Up!* and *Sleepless
Children*.

Also by Dr David Haslam

The Mothercare Guide For The Expectant Father
Travelling With Children
Parent Stress
Sleepless Children
Eat It Up!

Contents

Acknowledgements

I could not have written this book without the advice and help of a great many people. I simply cannot mention them all individually here, but I would particularly like to thank the many members of the Eating Disorders Association who wrote to me about their experiences. Their individual stories form the backbone of this book, which hopes to share something of the experience of bulimia. I promised them absolute confidentiality so that they could be completely open with me, and I have edited out any aspects of their stories which could identify them, as well as changing their names. My thanks to them all, whether I have quoted them or not.

I also wish to thank John Allen for his valuable advice on many aspects of psychological treatments, and the magnificent team in the library at Hinchingbrooke Hospital in Huntingdon for their assistance with my research into the medical literature. In addition, I am indebted to Dr Sîan Coker, who provided many valuable research papers, and to both Sarah Hannigan and Carole Blake.

I am especially grateful to Dr Chris Freeman, Consultant Psychiatrist at the Royal Edinburgh Hospital, for his permission to reproduce much of the Eating Diary used in his unit, and also the 'Principles of Normal Eating' quoted in Chapter 20.

HRH The Princess of Wales gave me great encouragement during the writing of this book, and I am most grateful to her both for this and for giving me permission to reproduce her speech to the International Conference on Eating Disorders

'93, given at Kensington Town Hall in April 1993.

Finally, may I thank Barbara, my wife, for her encouragement of my writing. Long hours spent at the word processor are more than a little anti-social, and I really do appreciate her support.

Preface

The symptoms of bulimia vary enormously, as do the problems that can result. The opening chapters of this book examine these, going on to look at the causes, and the different treatments that are currently available. Much of the final section of the book consists of a very positive self-help plan that enables people with bulimia to begin to eat normally again.

Throughout the book I have tended to refer to people with bulimia as 'she'. This is simply because there are many more female sufferers than male, and to write 'she or he' every time would be clumsy. I hope male sufferers will forgive me for I have devoted a specific chapter to your particular problems.

While writing the book I have assumed that you, the reader, have bulimia, as I felt this would have a more powerful and direct appeal. To this end I often refer to 'your' symptoms. If you are not a sufferer, there is a specific chapter which looks at the special needs and problems of families and friends; nevertheless all of the book should be of real interest and value to you.

Introduction

Jane is an airline hostess. Now aged twenty-seven, she developed bulimia just two years ago. She describes the start of the problem:

> I used to be quite heavy, about ten stone and I am only five foot three. I was this weight when I joined the airline, and was horrified when I saw myself on an airline video. It made me think for the first time that I was really fat. Before this, I had thought I was a bit plump, but it had never really bothered me. I developed this fixation about losing weight, so started the Rosemary Conley 'Hip and Thigh Diet', and very slowly and sensibly lost the weight. I got down to eight stone, and everyone remarked on how much better I looked. I started to get a lot more interest from the opposite sex, and I felt good in clothes I had never dared wear before. I even became much more confident with men. In the past I had never really bothered because no one ever showed any real interest in me.
>
> I don't recall exactly what happened to me to bring on the sudden change in my life. I wanted to be thin, I wanted to be protected, I wanted to be liked. I remember times that I looked in the mirror and hated what I saw, thinking I was fat and putting on weight. Slimness meant everything to me. The bulimia seemed to come on slowly. I remember going out for a meal, and then feeling guilty, and not wanting to put

on any weight, so I would take myself off to vomit.

I spend time away from home in different hotels, going out with the rest of the crew for meals. I knew that I would have to throw up, so I would take a toothbrush and toothpaste with me everywhere, with fresh make-up to touch up with after the vomiting made my eyes water.

One morning I was operating a flight from Aberdeen to Norwich, then on to Amsterdam. I had taken some cereal and skimmed milk for my breakfast, which I planned to have with some black coffee. During the flight I decided to eat a breakfast that had been put on board for the passengers – we had plenty left over. I then went on to eat four whole cooked breakfasts. These consisted of eggs, bacon, mushrooms, beans and sausage. I then had three bread rolls, two croissants, and countless pieces of toast. I just couldn't seem to stop, and I didn't really understand what was going on. I went to the toilet at the back of the aircraft and brought all of this up.

At Norwich I ate ten biscuits and six packets of peanuts. On the flight over to Amsterdam I ate the flight crew meal, three passenger meals, and more biscuits. I vomited all of this as well. As soon as it was over I needed to eat more. When I got home I had a cake, a dish of breakfast cereal, a family-sized block of ice cream, and then had to go to the shops to buy chocolate. I felt possessed. I couldn't control myself. I knew then that I really did need help.

Jane's story is not unusual. She wanted to be successful and popular, and she became obsessed with food. Her eating became totally out of control. She felt guilty, and stupid, wicked and depressed, and she even began to feel suicidal.

And she looked just fine.

None of her family knew of her problem. The aircrews with whom she worked thought she was the life and soul of the party, a happy-go-lucky member of the team. She didn't look too thin and she didn't look too fat. Until she plucked up the courage to talk, even her boyfriend knew nothing about her bulimia.

And when she did talk, they too felt shocked and astonished, worried and guilty. They did not know what to say, or how to help. They couldn't imagine anyone eating these quantities, or making themselves vomit. They didn't know how to begin to care for Jane, and this despair made them feel even worse.

Bulimia is a tragedy for the individual, and for her family and friends. But it can be helped. Understanding ways of coping with the problem will help you, and those around you. Whether you are a sufferer, or are worried about a friend or relative, it's important to realise that you are not alone. Many people feel just as you do, as you will see through their experiences. Don't despair; the outlook can be very positive indeed.

Jane's story is not at all unusual. As she said, 'The feelings that I encountered during my days of uncontrolled bulimia can only be described as being totally out of control, stricken by panic, disgusted by my body and my weakness. However, the things that helped me were knowing that I was not alone in the world with my misery, and also the love and support of my family and friends – who showed me nothing but kindness – and finding out as much about the condition as I could.'

If you suffer from bulimia, this book will provide a wealth of information about the condition, about the people who can help you and the ways in which you can help yourself, and it will attempt to clarify some of the explanations of why bulimia occurs.

If you are the relative or friend of a sufferer, I will explain what the problem involves, some of the reasons why it happens, the types of treatment that are available, the best ways in which you can help someone with bulimia. By understanding the condition, you will be less frightened by it, less disgusted and critical, and more tolerant. It may not be possible to put yourself in the shoes of the bulimia sufferer, but you can come close. As another sufferer told me, 'The non-bulimic will never, ever understand the paradoxical feelings of success, failure, punishment and reward that this way of life can give rise to. Eating disorders,' she went on, 'are insanity. You will never occupy my soul and experience that insanity. You will never know the relief I feel at having accepted myself and grown stronger. You will never understand the grief that I felt initially, knowing that I had to give up what had become my way of life in order to live at all. Eating disorders are psychological and chaotic. And outsiders will never fully comprehend this fact, just as I can never communicate it effectively enough.'

The many sufferers from bulimia to whom I have spoken have all shared this sense of being alone, and of being different. However, they are almost all remarkably good at sharing their feelings, and this sharing can only make life easier for themselves and others. If you suffer from bulimia and have never told anyone; if you are reading this book secretly, I hope you will read the words of many fellow sufferers and say, 'Yes – that's me! I feel like that.' Realising that you have bulimia, and that you are not alone with your feelings and fears, are the first and most important steps along the road to recovery.

T

1

A Definition of Bulimia

Twenty years ago, bulimia did not appear to exist. Today, almost everyone has heard of the condition. Magazines devote pages to articles and features on bulimia, newspapers speculate about whether film stars or others in the public eye might be sufferers. Bulimia, or to give it its full medical name, bulimia nervosa, has become almost acceptable. While this greater openness must be an excellent development, there are those who worry that bulimia might even have become fashionable. They worry that there could be a flipside to all this greater openness, in that more people might be tempted to try it. Indeed, some evidence of this sort of copy-cat behaviour exists.[1] This only becomes a danger, however, if bulimia is portrayed as an easy way to eat all you want and stay slim. As every sufferer will tell you, nothing could be further from the truth. I have no fear that this book might encourage anyone to become bulimic. The painful facts, the risks, and the long-term problems which can result will not be hidden.

The first classic text on eating disorders was published in 1974. In it, the author, Hilde Bruch, did not really discriminate between bulimia and anorexia. She stated that some anorexic women make themselves vomit, but did not discuss the existence of people with bulimia alone – those with characteristics quite different to anorexia nervosa.[2]

Many people now believe that eating disorders have

been in existence for centuries, certainly varying in the exact symptoms and social acceptability, but nevertheless recognisable as the conditions we know today. However, the very first mention of bulimia nervosa, the strict medical name for this condition, appeared in 1979 in a paper by Professor Gerald Russell of the Royal Free Hospital in London. The name 'bulimia' itself was apparently suggested by another doctor, Patrick Campbell, and derives from the Greek words 'bous' (ox) and 'limos' (hunger) – the appetite of an ox.[3]

In this original paper, bulimia was described as being an 'ominous variant' of anorexia nervosa. Again the author failed to consider the possibility that the conditions might be quite separate and distinct. He wrote, 'It would be premature to think of the disorder as constituting a distinct syndrome. It will still be seen as related to anorexia nervosa.' While much of this original paper was astonishingly accurate, even viewed from the perspective of years of later detailed research, this claim is no longer true. Bulimia is totally different from anorexia. Some people may suffer from both in their lifetime, but one does not seem to cause the other. So, as recently as 1979, knowledge of the condition was in its infancy.

Just fourteen years later, in April 1993, every single British daily newspaper devoted acres of newsprint to the Princess of Wales' speech on bulimia at a conference on eating disorders. This important speech contained many powerful images. As she said, 'I have it on very good authority that the quest for perfection our society demands can leave the individual gasping for breath at every turn. This pressure inevitably extends into the way we look.'

She went on to say, 'From the beginning of time the human race has had a deep and powerful relationship with food – if you eat you live, if you don't you die. Eating food has always been about survival, but also about caring for and nurturing the ones we love. However, with the added stresses of modern life, it has now become an expression of how we feel about ourselves and how we want others to feel about us.

'Eating disorders, whether anorexia or bulimia, show how individuals can turn the nourishment of the body into a painful attack on themselves, and they have at the core a far deeper problem than mere vanity. And, sadly, eating disorders are on the increase at a disturbing rate, affecting a growing number of men and women, and a growing number of children, too.'

Later in her speech she referred to some of the theories that have been put forward to explain bulimia. She acknowledged that 'our knowledge of eating disorders is still in its infancy. But it seems from those I've spoken to that the seeds of this disease may lie in childhood and the self-doubts and uncertainties that accompany adolescence. From early childhood many have felt they were expected to be perfect but didn't feel they had the right to express their true feelings to those around them – feelings of guilt, of self-revulsion and low personal esteem, creating in them a compulsion to "dissolve like a disprin" and disappear.'

The Princess of Wales' speech referred to the condition as a sufferer's 'shameful friend'. She said that 'by focusing their energies on controlling their bodies, they had found a refuge from having to face the more painful issues at the centre of their lives. A way of coping, albeit destructively and pointlessly, but a way of coping with a situation they were finding unbearable. An expression of how they felt about themselves and the life they were living.'

In talking about this 'shameful friend', the Princess of Wales opened the door for others to talk about their experiences. A number of celebrities came forward to say that they too had suffered from bulimia, including actress Jenny Seagrove, who was reported as saying, 'It got to the stage where I thought I was going to kill myself.'[4] Others who have been reported as having bulimia include Margot Hemingway, who was bulimic from the age of twelve, when she felt considerable pressure to be a 'perfect child', and Jane Fonda, who was also quoted as saying, 'It began

9

when I was twelve years old and at boarding school. I loved to eat, but I wanted to be thin. It wasn't long before I was bingeing and purging fifteen to twenty times a day.'[5]

In an interview with the film magazine, *Empire*, Andie MacDowell, star of *sex lies and videotape*, *Green Card* and *Groundhog Day*, said that she struggled with her appearance: 'I am in a constant struggle to keep the weight off. If I put on, say, twelve pounds, people will tell me that I am too fat. Would they do that to a man? Never! I have to have a flat stomach, perfect legs and skinny arms or I'll be considered fat.' The interviewer then asked if she'd ever been anorexic. Andie's reply was intensely honest. 'I was never anorexic,' she said. 'I wanted to be bulimic. I tried to make myself throw up and I just could not. I stuck my fist down my throat and nothing happened. I would have been bulimic if I could have been.'[6]

Just a very short time ago, these high-profile and highly publicised case histories would have been unheard of and almost unthinkable. Thankfully, times have changed, and people are now being more honest.

It wasn't always like this. Much of actress Lynn Redgrave's autobiography deals with her struggle with bulimia. She writes of her 'Fat Ogre', the desperate drive to binge eat, and how she 'discovered an amazingly easy way out. I started throwing up.' At that time, bulimia had not been officially reported, and certainly did not have a name. As a result, for some considerable time she believed that she was probably the only person in the world who did this. She was therefore quite astonished when one day she met Gilda Radner, a comedian who had recently made a big name for herself on America's 'Saturday Night Live' and who suddenly confessed that she too was bulimic.[7]

Mercifully, no bulimic today needs to feel alone. Feeling frightened, worried, guilty, depressed and distressed is quite enough for anyone.

A Definition of Bulimia

What exactly is bulimia? To begin with, let's get the scientific and academic definitions out of the way. In 1980, the American Psychiatric Association produced an extraordinarily thorough document called the 'Diagnostic and Statistical Manual of Mental Disorders (Third Edition)'.[8] Known by the shorter name of 'DSM-III', this contains the most clear and precise definition of bulimia. Clear definitions are essential. In such a complex disorder, it is vital that researchers who are looking at the problem in different ways can be certain that they are comparing like with like.

The brief summary of bulimia in DSM-III states that 'the essential features are binge eating accompanied by an awareness that the eating pattern is abnormal, fear of not being able to stop eating voluntarily, and depressed mood and self-deprecating thoughts following the eating binges. The bulimic episodes are not due to anorexia nervosa or any known physical disorder.'

The strict diagnostic criteria, which have to be met if the diagnosis of bulimia is to be made, are as follows:

A   Recurrent episodes of binge eating (rapid consumption of a large amount of food in a discrete period of time, usually less than two hours).
B   At least three of the following:
- consumption of high-caloric, easily ingested food during a binge;
- inconspicuous eating during a binge;
- termination of such eating episodes by abdominal pain, sleep, social interruption, or self-induced vomiting;
- repeated attempts to lose weight by severely restrictive diets, self-induced vomiting, or use of cathartics or diuretics; and
- frequent weight fluctuations greater than ten pounds due to the alternate binges and fasts.

C   Awareness that the eating pattern is abnormal and fear of not being able to stop eating voluntarily.

D Depressed mood and self-deprecating thoughts following eating binges.
E The bulimic episodes are not due to anorexia nervosa or any known physical disorder.

This original definition of bulimia, which dates from 1980, did not specify how often binge eating should occur. However, the revised criteria, known as the 'DSM-III-R Criteria' and published in 1987, say that there must be at least two episodes of binge eating per week for at least three months.[9]

Although not strictly part of the definition given above, some specialists in eating disorders subdivide bulimia into four groups, which can be helpful as the outlook for each group can be different.

- *Type I* These people have no previous history of anorexia nervosa, and are not considered phobic about their weight.
- *Type II* These sufferers do have a previous history of anorexia nervosa, and have recovered to a normal weight.
- *Type III* This group consists of those who were very overweight, and used purging and other bulimic activities as a means of dieting. They are now back to a normal weight (as defined by their BMI) but their bulimia persists.
- *Type IV* Those who have other problems such as drug or alcohol abuse, episodes of self-harm (e.g., repeated overdoses or wrist slashing) and general personality problems. I will return to this kind of bulimia, called Multi-Impulsive Bulimia, in Chapter 2.

Finally, before we finish with the jargon and the medical complexities, be warned that 'DSM-IV' is in the pipeline. Possible changes to the current definition are under discussion, but it's unlikely to differ much from the one above. Most published papers have used the DSM-III-R definition, so I have chosen to stick with this one. And there are even some specialists in eating disorders who suggest that splitting up the various types of eating disorder into different diagnoses is not helpful, but this is something I will return to in Chapter 13, when I look at the connections between bulimia and anorexia.

Important though this strict medical and psychiatric definition of the problem may be, what does it all really mean to the individual? Typically, and simply, the sufferer from bulimia has episodes of binge eating, followed by episodes of either purging, or strict dieting, fasting, or very vigorous exercise.

Binge eating normally consists of eating enormous quantities of food, typically food high in calories. Obviously binge eating is not an activity that can continue undetected, for considerable weight gain must follow excessive intake of calories. As sufferers normally binge in total secrecy, they then have to do something to reverse the effects of such a massive intake of calories.

Purging is usually achieved by self-induced vomiting; however, this is not the only way that bulimics try to get rid of all the extra calories. Some use high doses of laxatives; others abuse diuretic tablets. The effect of laxatives on calorie absorption is minimal. A few less calories may be absorbed but as most of the absorption of food occurs in the small intestine, and laxatives work on the large intestine, the effect is minimal. Laxatives don't work as a means of controlling 'real' weight. If someone has a massive clear out then they will weigh less – but this is entirely spurious weight loss. They weigh less because of having less weight of faeces in the bowel. And almost all bulimics come to learn that laxative abuse is useless, but when they stop they feel bloated, so they continue so as to avoid this bloated feeling. Again, this has nothing to do with weight loss.

Others who have binged try to reverse the harm they have done by periods of fasting, and some sufferers take up exercise to an excessive degree.

Perhaps the most extraordinary and extremely rare form of bulimia consists of blood letting. A report in the *British Journal of Psychiatry* in 1993 described two medical students and a junior doctor, all of whom had bulimia and had taken significant quantities of blood from themselves. One of these patients had taken over one litre of blood from herself and described, 'a relief of tension' which she recognised as being similar to the sensations she had felt after vomiting following a binge.[10]

In general, it is likely that purging, however performed, is the more harmful side of bulimia. Not only are there specific side-effects – which I will highlight in Chapter 5, but in a way the purging disguises and conceals the bingeing. If purging leaves the bingeing undetected, it is probably all the more likely that the whole cycle will be repeated.

When Eating Becomes a Problem

Eating should be one of life's pleasures. We should be able to enjoy eating without worrying endlessly about the effects that food will have on our body. Constant medical and health warnings about the dangers of eating some food or another have made many people neurotic about what they eat.

In recent years, milk and butter have been decreed too high in cholesterol, salt is blamed for high blood pressure, eggs carry a risk of causing salmonella, and as for white bread, health lobbyists have trouble describing how awful it is. The foods in which we've grown up finding comfort have all made the hit list, a list based, primarily, on incomplete research and scare stories.

This is nonsense. There are individuals for whom certain foods can cause problems, but for most of us eating a sensibly balanced diet with a little of what we fancy, and nothing in excess, will cause us no harm at all.

In the late twentieth century, certain foods are considered 'good' while others are 'bad'. Advertising campaigns for foods like cream cakes carry slogans such as 'naughty . . . but nice'. Food and guilt have been made allies. Food is no longer simply an enjoyable means of nourishment. When we have had a bad day, how many of us give ourselves a treat of some usually 'forbidden' food? When I've finished this chapter, I will have an extra cup of coffee, and probably a chocolate biscuit. Nothing to do with hunger. Everything to do with psychology. And entirely normal.

In bulimia all the normality has gone, and yet it is probably simply the extreme far end of the psychological spectrum that allows me my chocolate biscuit. Food is one of the most powerful rewards. Denial of food is one of the greatest punishments. And it is from this background that so many eating disorders stem.

No one ever has an entirely perfect diet, but there are three major and significant problems with eating that can arise. These are bulimia, anorexia nervosa and compulsive overeating. I will deal with some of the differences between bulimia and anorexia in Chapter 13, but there are some obvious similarities. In both conditions, the sufferer is preoccupied with food, dieting, their weight, and with being the right size and shape. A significant number of bulimia sufferers have previously suffered from anorexia, and people in both groups tend to feel extremely uncomfortable if they have to eat in public.

However, there are two main differences between these conditions. People with anorexia are always underweight, while those with bulimia can be any weight at all. In addition, people with anorexia almost always deny that they have a problem, sometimes even to themselves. Bulimics deny the problem to others but are all too aware of it personally. The typical sufferer from bulimia has family and friends who are completely oblivious to the problem, while she suffers in lonely isolation. Almost the exact opposite applies in anorexia nervosa: the family is well aware of the problem and the sufferer denies that it exists.

Almost everyone feels occasional guilt following an episode of over-indulgence. In bulimia the entire emotional response is quite different. Not only does the problem occur repeatedly, but the sufferer feels out of control, and intensely guilty and frightened. Many normal people will do a bit more exercise to right the damage of holiday eating; or, perhaps, cut down on fatty foods for a period of time. The onset of regular purging means that the problem is of quite different magnitude. As one bulimia sufferer noted with remarkable clarity, 'normal people who regret eating something simply shrug their shoulders and get on with life. I feel utterly compelled to correct the mistakes I have made. And this compulsion takes over my life.'

Understanding Bulimia

In the Introduction I quoted one bulimic who said, 'The non-bulimic will never, ever understand the paradoxical feelings of success, failure, punishment and reward that this way of life can give rise to.' However, there are ways that families and friends can try to understand what is going on in the bulimic's mind and body.

It is essential not to over-simplify the situation. Unsympathetic non-sufferers often say, 'They are just being greedy. They overeat, then feel guilty and vomit to get rid of the calories. Why can't they just control themselves in the first place?' What may seem a simple answer often disguises an ignorance of the reasons why people behave as they do.

Bernice is a 29-year-old accountant who wrote to me about her bulimia.

> I first realised that I suffered from bulimia when I was twenty-three years old. My brother had just got married, and my sister had got engaged. They were both younger than me, and while thrilled for them, I suppose I felt a bit left out. I'd just started a new job, and had arranged to go out for a meal with a girlfriend. I got home from work and everyone was out, so I had a biscuit. And then another, and another. I also ate jam straight from the jar, raisins, honey, cheese, ham, bread, chocolate. I stuffed anything and everything that I could lay my hands on into my mouth. My heart was pounding very loudly, and I ate very quickly, jumping from one food to another, but never eating all of anything. If I ate all except one biscuit in a packet I thought Mum and Dad would never notice.
>
> I started crying and felt disgusted with myself. I couldn't stop crying and I felt so awful. I phoned the doctor and made an appointment. The receptionist

could barely make out what I was saying as I was crying so hard.

Dad then came home and found me crying. I told him what I'd eaten, and he said, 'Why don't you just stop yourself?' but that's just it. I couldn't stop myself.

Bulimics will understand exactly how Bernice felt. Non-bulimics may feel mystified, just like Bernice's father. However, if you want to understand bulimia, you really do need to consider three quite separate aspects of the problem. These are:

- the eating behaviour – how the bulimic eats and purges;
- how the bulimic perceives herself and her world; and
- how the bulimic copes with her emotions.

Psychologists describe these three aspects of behaviour as the behavioural, the cognitive and the emotional. It is essential to understand all three if you want to begin to appreciate the torment of having bulimia.

If we look at Bernice's case, it is possible to unravel these three strands of understanding.

Behavioural

Bernice has described exactly what she did. Later, she went on to say, 'Over the next few weeks my eating got worse. I'd pig out every day, buying chocolate bars and hiding the wrappers, and always eating when Mum and Dad were in another room. Then I'd drink syrup of figs straight from the bottle. I'd swallow a handful of Nylax tablets every day. The laxatives didn't seem to work, so I'd up the doses I was taking . . .'

Bernice's bingeing and purging are absolutely typical, and give us a clear understanding of *what* she did. However, it is even more important to begin to understand why.

Cognitive

The way that Bernice felt about herself was absolutely

clear. As she said, 'I started crying and felt disgusted with myself.' She felt totally out of control, guilty and even wicked. Very many sufferers from bulimia believe that their size and shape is affecting their lives. One said, 'I was quite convinced that I'd be happier if I was slim.'

In Chapter 7 I will return to the important effect of society's attitude to slimness, but in the meantime ask yourself what all those slimming magazines are really selling. Happiness. Look at the before and after photographs of the slimmers. The overweight are never smiling quite as broadly as the slim. But whatever the advertisements say, slimness does not guarantee happiness, and it never will.

Emotional

When Bernice first started bingeing she was fed up. Depressed. Miserable. Her self-esteem was already low, after her brother's wedding and the subsequent engagement of her sister. As the bulimia progressed she became more and more guilty and afraid.

Eventually she saw a community psychiatric nurse, and wrote, 'And then, for the first time, I began to realise just how depressed I felt. I met her every week, and started to feel better about myself. From psychotherapy I can now see how all through my childhood I tried so hard to please my Dad, and yet never once felt that I did have his approval. I had to be perfect, and when I decided not to go to university I felt I'd let him down.'

In later chapters I will return to some of the causes of bulimia, including complicated family problems like Bernice's. For now it is simply worth noting that nothing in bulimia is as simple as it seems. When Bernice's father asked why she couldn't stop herself, he was expressing his confusion and lack of understanding. After help from many individuals, Bernice is now fine. She explored and understands her emotions.

Bernice finished by saying, 'Now, I'm a very different

person. I feel all kinds of emotions now instead of keeping them in. I have met and married a wonderful man who knows about my bulimia and doesn't hide away from the things I went through. Moving away from home was difficult, but we coped. My advice to other sufferers – confide in a friend, and find a local group who can help you.'

If you are going to confide in a friend, or in your family, why not lend them this book when you have finished it? Simply hoping that bulimia will disappear will not work. Trying to understand what is happening is the first step of the path to recovery.

Suffering from Bulimia

As we have seen, people with bulimia suffer from two main groups of symptoms. Firstly, there is the compulsion to binge. Following this, the bulimic will attempt to un-do the damage, by either self-induced vomiting, the use of laxatives; or numerous other methods. In the next two chapters I will deal in considerable detail with both bingeing and purging, but before doing this it is worth examining some of the more general features of this condition.

If you suffer from bulimia, you are bound to recall all too clearly the first time that the problem reared its head. If you don't have bulimia yourself, you may wonder how it could possibly happen. How could anyone find themselves in this position?

How Does It Start?

Bulimia is predominantly a problem that starts in adolescence, with binge eating typically beginning between the ages of fourteen and twenty-four.[1] The seeds of the condition may be sown at a much younger age, even though very few sufferers actually develop symptoms in childhood.

Patricia, whose story is not at all unusual, told me of her experiences:

> Since the age of twelve I can remember the daunting experience of not being able to get any clothes to fit me. It was a nightmare trying clothes on. I used to

feel angry, and annoyed that I was so fat. Indeed this dreaded word was used frequently within my family and school-day experiences. Family pressure was never ending:

'You're too fat.'

'Why don't you lose some weight?'

'You'd be much happier if you weren't fat.'

I experienced vicious teasing at school. Verbal and physical teasing made my school days miserable and non-productive. At the age of sixteen, my weight was twelve stone. I felt desperately unhappy and went on my first serious diet when I left home to go to college at sixteen. I managed to lose about two stone. I felt better, but the thought of getting obese again haunted me day and night. I bought my first packet of laxatives at sixteen, and I would occasionally make myself vomit, particularly after I had gorged myself. However, I hadn't yet discovered the nightmare of bingeing. That happened when I was twenty-two, studying at university, hoping to be a teacher.

Another bulimia sufferer told me, 'As far back as I can remember in childhood I had felt fat and frumpy. I turned to food for comfort for many years, and then tried dieting on many occasions, too. The big diet came when I was twenty. The beginning of the problem.'

In later chapters I will discuss the various theories about why bulimia occurs, but these feelings of inadequacy, of feeling fat and unattractive, are tremendously important. Obviously, not everyone who is teased about their weight develops an eating disorder, but bulimia frequently follows an obsession with dieting. It seems such an easy answer. Why bother to diet, if you can get rid of the calories quickly and simply? If it were simple, harmless and effective, bulimia would not be a problem, but dieting, and over-concern with dieting, can be very bad for your health.

Indeed, bulimia almost always begins with dieting and an overwhelming desire to lose or control one's weight. Sometimes it begins accidentally, with a natural vomit after an episode of bingeing. On other occasions, the sufferer may hear about it from friends, or articles, books or television. And everyone who starts with bulimia believes that she can control it. Like the use of drugs or alcohol, the user believes that he or she can be in control. But, sadly, the very people who are most likely to experiment with bingeing and purging, are almost certainly the same people who will have difficulty controlling the habit.

While there is a similarity with conditions like alcohol abuse – bulimics find it difficult to control their habit once it has started – it's essential to realise that *bulimia is not an addiction*. Even more fundamentally, people with alcohol problems can learn to cope without alcohol, but ex-bulimics can never ever manage without food. But alcohol, drug abuse and bulimia can all be a response to being depressed.

Sweets after school

The actual symptoms of bulimia rarely start in childhood, but there is little doubt that in everyone, whether bulimic or not, eating and the emotions are inextricably combined from the very earliest days. Feeding and eating are not just matters of mechanical refuelling. The child who doesn't eat properly, or refuses certain foods, causes his parents great concern. Almost all parents worry at times about what their child is or isn't eating, and as a source of concern, despair, guilt and anger it is almost without equal. After all, parents know that diet is vitally important, and often both the quality and quantity of food that their child will eat differs from their own ideas of good nutrition.

Parents despair that children sometimes seem to go out of their way to reject 'healthy' foods, seeming, automatically, to choose 'junk'. Parents can spend hours cooking a meal, only to have the children turn up their noses and refuse to eat it. Worry about food refusal is very common. In one American study, around one in five three-year-olds were described as having a very poor appetite, and more than one in ten had very finicky tastes and ate an extremely limited diet.[2] In the UK, John and Elizabeth Newson found that 42 per cent of the parents of four-year-olds in Nottingham were concerned about their child's eating habits.[3]

If feeding were simply a matter of letting appetite dictate how much one eats, then parents would not go through all the efforts that they do to encourage their child to eat more. Most parents will try the trick of 'choo-choo-training' an extra spoonful of food into their reluctant child's mouth. 'Just one more spoonful,' they plead. They even offer rewards for finishing a plate of food. And look at the restaurants that cater for children, such as Little Chefs and Happy Eaters. Almost all offer a lollipop or sweet to the child who clears his or her plate. A child who eats more than he or she wants is praised.

Food is used as a reward in other ways too. How many parents say to their children, 'If you are good at the doctor's I'll give you some sweets'? How many greet their children at the end of the day with sweets after school? How many use sweets, crisps or biscuits to keep their child quiet while shopping, or in the car? And how many withhold food as a punishment: 'If you misbehave, you can't have any sweets'?

It is not surprising that food becomes so important to us, and that we all grow up seeing certain foods as a reward. For a small group of people, this use of food as a reward can get out of hand later in life, leading to bulimia.

Indeed, even though bulimia itself in childhood is very rare, it is all too obvious that some of the psychological links between eating and the emotions have been present with us all since we were very small children.

It is clear that food and feeding comes to be far more important in a child's life than simply as nourishment. Even in infancy parents may offer food to calm an unhappy baby. Hilde Bruch, who was, as we discussed earlier, one of the first researchers to look at bulimia, has hypothesised that this is the way that the child uses food to satisfy many needs as well as hunger. Indeed, from a psychodynamic viewpoint, food can come to stand for love or power, or can express rage and hate, and can even become a substitute for sex.[4]

23

Early Onset Bulimia

As we have seen, the majority of sufferers from bulimia develop the problem between the ages of fifteen and twenty-four, but there is a small sub-group who develop the problem much earlier.

One study looked at the difference between people with 'early onset bulimia', and those who developed the problem later. No significant differences were found in eating behaviour between the two groups, but deliberate self-harm occurred more commonly in the younger group, and there was also a trend towards more depression among their relatives. Interestingly, the young group had been exposed to more social and domestic stresses, the result, for instance of the family moving home, or a parent losing a job.[5]

Occasionally, the causes of childhood bulimia are even more dramatic. Julia works as a holiday company representative, but her early years were a nightmare.

> I first started making myself sick at the age of seven years, and it went on and off for years. Sometimes I was fine for months at a time, and then it would all begin again. I was sexually abused from the age of five to sixteen years by our next-door neighbour. When I was seven years, he first made me have oral sex, and that's when I first began being sick. Everything was done in secret, and no one knew. When I was seventeen years old I could cope no more, and I took my first overdose.

Julia's story may be unusual, but it is almost certainly not unique. Later in this book I will return to the topic of sexual abuse; if your bulimia started when you were abused you can feel reassured that you are not alone. Do try and tell someone. If you don't know where to turn, your family doctor will treat everything you say in complete confidence, and will be able to direct you to appropriate counselling and help.

Multi-Impulsive Bulimia

This tendency towards self-harm that can occur in bulimia, particularly in those with an early onset of the problem, may be part of a condition known as 'multi-impulsive bulimia'. For these patients the eating problem is only one of a number of similar problems that disrupt, and even endanger, their lives.

It was recognised some time ago that bulimic patients who also abuse alcohol do less well in treatment than those with bulimia alone.[6] These bulimics with an alcohol problem also tended to show one or more other behavioural characteristics which were self-damaging, such as abuse of drugs, repeated overdoses, sexual disinhibition, and so on. Strict diagnostic criteria have been suggested for this condition of multi-impulsive bulimia.[7]

First of all, the bulimia will be associated with any one or more of the following behaviours:

- alcohol abuse;
- 'street' drug abuse;
- multiple overdoses;
- repeated mutilation – such as wrist-cutting;
- sexual disinhibition; and
- shoplifting.

You may find it curious that an activity like shoplifting appears on this list, but the second criterion for diagnosis of this condition is that each of these behaviours will be associated with a feeling of being out of control. The sufferer does not deliberately choose to go into a store to steal a blouse, cassette or whatever. Instead the act is impulsive, as out-of-control as the frightening over-eating of bulimia.

Sufferers from multi-impulsive bulimia tend to fluctuate between these patterns of behaviour. At any one time one of these particular behaviour characteristics will be most noticeable. At other times it will be another. Inevitably people in this group tend to have a very low sense of self-esteem, and when they do manage to control these behaviours, they tend to become either intensely depressed, intensely angry, or both.

The interchangeable symptoms mean that this group are particularly hard for therapists to treat. If, as an example, the sufferer gets help for her bulimia at an appropriate clinic, and her eating becomes under control, the binge-eating and vomiting may well stop. However, at the same time she may then move on to drug abuse, or self-harm – like cutting her wrists or other forms of self-mutilation.

It is fair to say that this particular group does tend to be more emotionally disturbed than other bulimics, and they tend to do less well with treatment. If you, or someone you care for, does seem to fall into this category then it is almost certainly necessary to seek help as an in-patient at a specialist unit. Your doctor should be able to put you in touch with a suitable centre, or contact one of the groups given in Appendix A, pages 216–17.

The self-help and other treatment techniques that I will be discussing in the second half of this book will not be sufficient to unravel the complex problems of this small sub-group of bulimia sufferers. Treatment really does need to be intensive, and it has been proposed that each patient has an individual psychotherapist in order to help work through the causes of this distressing problem, and to enable her to gain insight into why she is the way she is.[8]

These patients are also encouraged to develop new ways of dealing with their feelings and particularly their inter-personal difficulties, and this is an area that all bulimia sufferers need to consider.

Bingeing

Almost anyone who has ever been on a diet will understand one of the main aspects of binge eating, even if they have never suffered from bulimia. Let us say you are on a strict calorie-controlled diet, and have had a carefully chosen breakfast, with black coffee, orange juice and a small bowl of cereal. You arrive at work to find that it is a colleague's birthday. During your break she produces a delicious, cream-filled chocolate cake. It would be rude to refuse, so you have a small slice.

And at this point a voice inside you says, 'Well, you've blown it now. There was no point in being careful, was there? Forget the diet for today. You've eaten too much already. You can always start again tomorrow.'

And so you have a second slice of cake, and a large lunch, and a glass or two of wine in the evening, and you keep saying to yourself, 'There's no point in dieting today anyway. I might as well enjoy myself, and start my diet again tomorrow.'

Logical thought tells you that all this is nonsense. There is nothing magical about starting a diet tomorrow, or next week, or any other time. If you are on a diet then every extra calorie matters. If you've had the birthday cake today, eating more and more of other foods will simply make things worse. But almost everyone who has ever tried to diet will have faced these thoughts at times.

This description is not an attempt to belittle the dreadful

strain that bingeing in bulimia can cause. It is an attempt to give the non-bulimic an introduction to how the dreadful spiral of bingeing can occur. The binge eating of someone with bulimia can be frightening and uncontrollable. The sufferer feels guilty and disgusted with herself, but quite unable to stop.

Binge eating is quite different from severe hunger. In a typical episode of bingeing, the bulimic will eat an abnormally large amount of food, simultaneously losing control over what she is eating. She's not hungry. She doesn't feel full while the binge is going on. All the normal sensations of control which most of us feel simply seem to disappear.

The amount of food taken in can be quite astonishing. Typically it tends to be the sort of food that one would not eat on a calorie-controlled diet. Indeed a binge is often the exact opposite of what most people consider a 'diet'. And the loss of control can be frightening, overpowering and almost unimaginable. In one study of 316 bulimic women, it was found that most of the women binged at least once each day. This usually occurred in the evening, and the binges averaged 4800 calories. One bulimia sufferer said to me, 'I know the amounts I eat may seem remarkable, but it never seems to matter as I know I'm going to be sick anyway.' In this study the range was between 1000 calories, and an almost unimaginable 55,000 calories. The majority of the foods eaten in the binge were sweet or salty carbohydrates.[1] However, other research has suggested that food consumed during binges is just as likely to contain fat or protein as it does carbohydrate. The really decisive factor governing what foods are eaten is simply which foods are available.

For some people, a binge will mean eating whatever is available in the kitchen cupboards – the bread and jam, crisps, cereal, biscuits or cakes. For others, the compulsion to eat everything and anything can be overwhelming, to an extent that many people will find incomprehensible.

Sally, a 21-year-old bank worker, graphically described her own frightening experiences:

Whenever I felt really down or desperate I would binge. I felt empty emotionally and would feed myself. But the guilt after stuffing my face was so great, and I could not stand the food being inside of me. I hated anything and everything inside me, whether it was greasy chips or a healthy apple! I hate to be sick, but the bingeing got more and more out of control, and I spent a huge amount of my savings – all on food. I would eat anything and everything, but always, always in private. I'd eat loaves of bread, butter, jam, large cream cakes (even if they were still frozen), yoghurts, chocolates, crisps, buns, anything. It got to the point where I could not control it at all. I would even hang around the kitchen after supper until everyone had left the room, and then I would take all the food thrown away into the bin and stuff it into my face as if I'd not seen food for weeks! I didn't taste the food. I just stuffed it in as quickly as I possibly could. I'd then go out in the dark and I'd go down the public street bins, looking for food. I have been a vegetarian for about seven years. But on a binge I would eat anything – even meat, although I never bought meat myself. But if there was meat in the bin – I'd eat it. I ate such incredible food – frozen, raw, stale, mouldy. At the worst stage of my life I was making myself sick up to seventy times in a day.

Sally's description gives some hint of the sheer compulsion that takes over during an episode of bingeing. She is certainly not alone. Charlotte, an Oxford University student, particularly highlights the isolation and loneliness that sufferers feel.

It was worst during my first two years at university, and the main thing was the secrecy – the total isolation. Other people saw me as competent, caring, good at organising things, good at my subject and my music, and always ready to listen if they had a problem. (I must add that this was someone else's description of me. I've never felt anything that positive.) It was essential that they never ever should see the other side of me – the disgusting greedy side that could spend up to £30 on a binge, and not even on nice food, spending hours eating and vomiting, sticking a spoon or toothbrush down my throat, taking anything up to 200 laxatives a day, desperately trying to make myself feel clean again. If anyone saw this, I felt sure they would simply run away in disgust.

The ease with which bulimia can be kept secret is often quite surprising. Because bulimics are frequently a normal weight, no one suspects that anything is wrong with them. Husbands, boyfriends, parents and family can all be completely unaware of the nightmare of bingeing and purging.

Gloria lives at home with her parents. While they are now aware that she has a problem with bulimia, they have little idea of exactly what she is going through. Her account gives some idea of the depression that she feels.

Last weekend I had yet another bad bulimic attack. On Saturday night, during the night I woke and made straight for the kitchen. I got the keys of the kitchen from Mum (she keeps the kitchen door locked over night to keep me out) with the excuse that I wanted a glass of milk. I started to binge and felt so frightened that I took four of Dad's sleeping tablets to make me sleep. Needless to say I slept well into Sunday afternoon.

When I woke up I felt so rotten that all I could think of was having a binge to help me cope. I made the excuse to Mum that I had a really sore throat and asked her if she would go to my sister who lives fourteen miles away and get a bottle of 'Night Nurse' for me. Mum agreed to do this and Dad went out too. That was it. I raided the kitchen eating absolutely everything in sight – pies, biscuits, crisps, even uncooked meat. The result was inevitable. I was sick. I went back to bed. It goes on like this every day. I must change. I want to change. But I never do.

Bulimia can be helped, but as a sufferer you are probably feeling real desperation until you find that help. Another bulimic student voices this feeling,

I feel like I'm still on this yo-yo. I go for a couple of days without bingeing and then something breaks and

I just give in. That's it then until I hit the point where I just want to cry because I'm so fed up with it (and this phase can last anywhere between a couple of weeks and a couple of months). One of my incentives at the moment is 'Well, I can't stop myself from bingeing a lot of the time, but I can get through the day by eating very little.' I know it's not a very healthy attitude, but I do know it's only temporary. I just remind myself to take it one day at a time.

The great majority of binge eaters try to counteract their intermittently excessive calorie intake by vomiting or purging. However a minority simply alternate the bingeing with strict dieting. 'As long as I didn't eat anything at all,' wrote Maureen, one former sufferer, 'I felt all right. But, the moment I ate anything I felt as if all my dieting had been wasted. I just went wild – eating everything in sight. I had no sense of perspective. Letting just a few calories past my lips made me feel as if dieting was pointless. And if dieting was pointless and I was going to end up fat, I might as well go the whole hog. So I did. Literally.'

Another sufferer told me that her binges were almost always of apples. 'I knew apples were all right if I was on a diet. Not many calories. Good for me. Full of vitamins. That sort of thing. So I would eat up to twenty at a time. I sometimes thought my stomach would burst, but I simply couldn't stop myself.'

Geraldine is a thirty-year-old mother of two who suffers with bulimia. She sent me a list of what she ate during her last episode of severe bingeing. If I had not heard of such extraordinary quantities from so very many people, I would judge them to be physically impossible. But they are all too possible for the person with bulimia:

> one chocolate cake
> two bags of cheese and onion potato crisps
> one wholemeal loaf
> half a stale sliced white loaf
> one family-sized can of salted peanuts
> two chocolate bars
> half a box of breakfast cereal with sugar and milk

one can of whipped pudding
one can of instant custard
one packet of sliced ham
one carton of double cream
at least one litre of cola
one packet of biscuits

Not only is the calorie input from such a binge quite remarkable – probably near to ten thousand calories – but the cost is considerable, too. Bingeing can be both expensive and dangerous. Indeed, perhaps the most dangerous episode of bingeing that I came across in my research was a diabetic lady who on one single occasion ate an astonishing one hundred and thirty chocolate bars. She worked in a cash and carry store where such quantities were to hand. Nevertheless, it is little wonder that after an experience like this she ended up in coma, in hospital.

While most bulimia sufferers can often manage to keep the problem a secret, a few leave a real mess, with cans, jars, plates and dishes spread about for everyone to see. The actual time it takes to binge varies considerably. A single bingeing episode may last from only a few minutes to hours, or even a day or more. Approximately one in three binge eaters have specific times of the week when they binge – often when they know they are going to be alone.

It is also important to realise that there are degrees of binge eating, and that bingeing may not always involve eating enormous quantities. For some people a binge may simply involve eating a food that they feel they should not. This could be no more than a single chocolate bar, or cheese sandwich. These binges have been described as 'subjective binges' and while they are obviously less dramatic, they can still be very distressing.

Why Do Binges Occur?

It is relatively unusual for actual hunger to trigger off a binge. As some of these quotations from bulimia sufferers have shown, an individual episode of bingeing may be triggered off by other isolated events or feelings. Classified simply, these may be linked to mood, to diet and/or to body image.

Mood changes are the most common trigger. Frequently the individual feels depressed, lonely, tense, frightened, angry or simply unhappy. As Sally said, 'Whenever I felt really down or desperate I would binge. I felt empty emotionally and would feed myself.' This is an extremely common experience, and may lead to a vicious circle: the bulimia makes you unhappy, and the unhappiness makes you bulimic.

For over ten years I have been using this concept of 'vicious circles' to help people understand their emotional problems.[2,3] The vicious circle of binge-eating is one of the simplest and the most powerful. This can be easily illustrated:

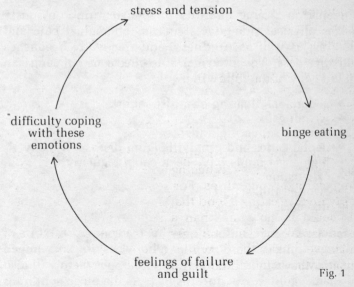

stress and tension

binge eating

feelings of failure
and guilt

difficulty coping
with these
emotions

Fig. 1

However, these emotional triggers are not the only reasons for attacks of bingeing. Thoughts or anxiety about food itself can be a problem. The person who has put herself on a diet may begin a binge if she feels she has transgressed and eaten something 'forbidden'. Indeed some people may feel irresistible temptation if they have access to so-called 'fattening' foods. As Jayne, another bulimic, said, 'Letting just a few calories past my lips made me feel as if dieting was pointless. And so I went the whole hog.' It has been estimated that over 90 per cent of bulimia sufferers often say that they have been overeating, and have usually put themselves on a strict diet before they started binge eating.

Finally, some triggers of bulimia may be linked to concern about body size, shape or appearance. 'If I'm that fat, what's the point in being careful?' Simply feeling fat or bloated may trigger off a 'What the hell?' attack of bingeing, as may the misery and depression involved in this episode of worsening self-esteem.

The After-effects of Bingeing

Bingeing on a large quantity of food or drink obviously causes physical side-effects such as abdominal pain and bloating, as well as tiredness, and frequently headaches and dizziness. The physical side-effects of bingeing can include any of the following:

- abdominal bloating and discomfort;
- weight gain;
- swollen salivary glands;
- dental caries and gingivitis (gum disease) if many high-sugar foods have been eaten regularly;
- exhaustion;
- swollen limbs; and
- dizziness and nausea.

Emotionally the sufferer may have a complex mixture of feelings. Initially there may be relief at having succumbed to the overwhelming temptation to eat, but there will also be shame, guilt, regret and disgust. As the binge continues there may be panic.

However, if bulimia only gave unpleasant sensations it would not be something that people would continue to do. Some people have suggested that bingeing on refined carbohydrates creates a sensation of being 'high' when the surge of sugar reaches the brain. People find that eating can calm them down, can be a pleasant way of passing the time, and may be relaxing. As discussed earlier, food is used as a reward from our earliest days, and someone who is down may reward themselves with a binge – an overdose of food. And some bulimics have a sensation of having punished the person they blame for their problems – a kind of 'Now see what you've made me do' mentality.

Nearly all bulimics will go through a period in which they try to resist their bingeing. Possible ways in which they might do this can include:

- buying as little food as possible, and not keeping food available in the house;
- being as frenetically active as possible, taking up every waking moment with activities – this could be socialising, doing hobbies, exercising or almost anything;
- telephoning friends when the urge to binge comes on;
- deliberately slowing the speed at which they eat food;
- keeping a jigsaw puzzle in the kitchen, so that every time she goes into the room to eat, she deliberately displaces her activity into putting more pieces in the pattern;
- eating more foods that they see as 'good' – e.g., fruit, vegetables and similar foods;
- resorting to drugs or alcohol which may ease the problem with bulimia by replacing it temporarily with another problem that will still need to be sorted out.

At the end of the day, some of these controlling behaviours may help temporarily, but as long as the underlying problems remain untackled, the urge to binge eat will continue. Following a large binge, the majority of bulimics will need to clear their system of all the extra calories that they have taken on board. The ways in which they can do this are dealt with in the next chapter.

Preventing Weight Gain

It goes without saying that someone who regularly binges on ten thousand calories, or who eats stale food or uncooked meat, cannot safely continue in this way without becoming grossly obese, unwell or both. For most bulimics the fear of becoming overweight is every bit as great as their love, or lust, for food.

There are a number of ways in which the sufferer from bulimia can attempt to reverse this excessive calorie intake. These include:

- very strict dieting;
- self-induced vomiting;
- laxative abuse;
- diuretic tablet abuse;
- excessive exercise – particularly jogging, playing squash, swimming or aerobics; and
- using amphetamine-based slimming tablets.

In one study of 316 patients with bulimia, the great majority of the women were using purging techniques to get rid of their excessive calorie intake. 81 per cent used self-induced vomiting and 63 per cent used laxative medication. Interestingly this particular study showed a significant delay of approximately one year between beginning bingeing and starting to purge.[1] However, in understanding bulimia it is vital to realise that, while purging usually starts as an attempt to control weight, the longer that the bulimia goes on, the more it is likely to become that person's chief way of dealing with emotion.

Bingeing and Fasting

> When I first began bingeing the answer seemed obvious. If I ate too much on one occasion, all I had to do was eat less on others. I even got a calorie counter and calculator. After a binge, I worked out how many meals I would have to miss before I could eat again. I did as much sport as I could. Using up more calories meant that I could eat a little more. But it all took my life over. I either seemed to be bingeing, or starving, or running. It all became too much. That was when I discovered how to make myself vomit.

Calorie counting and exercise are, of course, perfectly acceptable methods of controlling one's weight. Every sensible diet book explains that whether you lose or gain weight depends on the balance between the calories that are eaten and those that are burned off. If you eat as many calories as you use then your weight remains stable.

However sensible this can be, dieting and exercise can get out of control. It's like eating and bingeing. Everyone understands and accepts that there is nothing wrong with the occasional cream cake, eaten as a treat when one is feeling down. But, bingeing on twenty thousand calories in a sitting is harmful and undesirable. Similarly, eating virtually nothing for days on end is clearly a long way down the spectrum from the ordinary calorie-controlled diet.

A student dentist describes her relationship with food:

> When I was living at home I always bought diet foods, and tried to avoid eating with the family. But sadly my diets never really seemed to work. At least once every ten days they ended with an orgy of eating. This would leave me depressed. I promised myself that it wouldn't happen again, and the dieting became even stricter. All the next day I would starve. Indeed I once managed to go for nearly four days without

eating at all, but eventually I couldn't hang out any longer. Any food I had in my room would get eaten. I would also go swimming and play tennis as often as I could, and began to jog. I became worried that I had become addicted to exercise, but it did make me feel better and I suppose that helped.

Many bulimics seem to believe that it is their average calorie intake that matters. On a very simple level, if someone normally lives well on 2000 calories per day, they might think that a binge of 5000 calories, followed by four days eating just 250 calories would give the same total and be perfectly safe. While the arithmetic is correct, the metabolism does not agree.

Indeed, there is now plenty of evidence that repeated dieting – sometimes known as yo-yo dieting – can actually lead to weight gain.[2] Our bodies are designed to survive in adverse situations. If only a little food is entering the stomach, the body does not know that this is deliberate, and it becomes far more efficient metabolically. The body protects itself, slowing down the metabolism so that fewer calories are needed to maintain function and weight. Inevitably, when normal eating resumes, the body is still functioning with a slower metabolism, and weight gain can result. Dieting can actually cause weight gain. Indeed many non-bulimic frequent dieters find that the more they go on and off diets, the more easily they gain weight, and the heavier they become.

While some bulimics use diet to control their weight by fasting or strict calorie-counting, others do so by avoiding what they see as 'bad foods' – foods that are perceived as fattening. Unfortunately, as anyone who has ever dieted knows, the more you diet, the more you think about food. The more you think about food, the hungrier you get. And the hungrier you get, the more likely you are to binge. In a bulimia sufferer this binge can be wildly excessive. In the last chapter I discussed how an understanding of vicious circles can help your understanding of the causes and pressures of binge eating. The same applies equally to the effect of dieting. Indeed this particular vicious circle can mean that dieting actually worsens the frequency of binges.

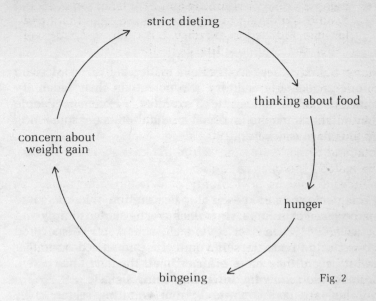

Fig. 2

Exercise

Exercise is obviously a sensible and healthy way to control weight gain, but even this can get out of hand. The bulimic who spends hours running, jogging, swimming, doing aerobics, or other sports may have the right intentions, but without tackling the other problems of bulimia no amount of exercise will be the answer.

Exercise works in two ways to control weight. Exertion obviously uses up calories, though in itself this is of minimal importance. Running for an hour would theoretically only work off a single chocolate biscuit, if it were not for the other effects on metabolism. There is now evidence that the metabolism is stimulated for several hours after exercise. In other words more calories are used up than are burnt off by the exercise alone.

In addition, exercise is known to help depression and

lift the mood,[3] it helps to prevent osteoporosis in women,[4] and obviously helps to keep the heart, lungs and muscles fit. Unfortunately, exercise becomes unhealthy if done too much. An individual can become addicted to running, working out, and so on to a quite obsessive degree. 'Fit' is not synonymous with 'healthy'.

And, sadly, there seems to be evidence that people who exercise regularly actually eat more than their sedentary neighbours.[5] In moderation, exercise is excellent. People with bulimia tend to find that moderation is not something that comes very naturally.

Self-induced Vomiting

This doctor provided a graphic description of her personal experience of bulimia; she tells how she started simply and effectively: 'When I was seventeen,' she wrote, 'I discovered that I could make myself vomit. I found I need no longer worry about the excess calories in all the food I had eaten, but I could rectify the binges by being sick.'[6]

This is a common perception; vomiting seems to be the answer to bingeing and worries about weight. Many bulimics almost feel a sense of euphoria when they discover that they can make themselves sick – a euphoria that fades rapidly when they find that the bingeing occurs more and more frequently. Later in this doctor's moving article, she described a binge, which all started with an overwhelming desire to eat cereals or breads: 'At some stage a point was reached after which I decided if I ate any more I would make myself vomit. Continuing to eat was then easy, as I knew none of the food would count later. I would spend half an hour sticking my fingers down my throat. Afterwards I would cry for a few hours.'

As we discussed earlier, the great majority of bulimics do make themselves vomit – usually in the toilet or bathroom where the noise of flushing, or running water, can disguise the sound of retching. The technique may be as simple as sticking one's fingers into the back of the throat, or else using the handle of a spoon, or a toothbrush, or even rolled-up paper. After a while, many women discover that they can induce vomiting by contracting the diaphragm and stomach muscles until food enters the oesophagus, and is vomited. For some it actually becomes as simple as pressing the hand against the upper abdomen.

Although some people vomit only once, many bulimics who use vomiting will repeat this up to ten or more times in an attempt to ensure that all the food has been cleared from the stomach. Some drink copious amounts of water and then vomit this, to wash out the stomach. Others start a binge with a particularly distinctive food, such as a tomato. Then, when they vomit, they will recognise this in the vomit, and know that they have cleared everything.

Surprisingly, despite frequent vomiting, bulimic women tend not to develop aversions to the taste of the foods that they eat and vomit. In addition, the food that is vomited is relatively undigested, which makes the taste nowhere near as noxious as the vomiting that we have all experienced during a stomach upset.

A very few bulimics have even resorted to swallowing a narrow rubber tube in order to wash out the contents of the stomach – the same technique that is used in hospital emergency departments to clear the stomachs of those who take overdoses. If anything illustrates the despair that bulimia can cause, it must surely be this – a harrowing form of self-punishment carried out in lonely secrecy.

Laxative Abuse

The logic behind laxative abuse is a rather ill-considered one. One patient expressed it this way: 'If I can get the food through my system quicker,' she said, 'there will be less time for the calories to be absorbed.' Various estimates suggest that three out of four bulimics will use laxatives at some time, and not only do the users believe that laxatives will prevent weight gain, they also find that purging does ease the bloated feeling that inevitably follows a binge.

Certainly laxatives can speed up peristaltic activity in the intestinal tract, and the idea of encouraging food to 'go through' rather than be absorbed is behind a number of diets, in particular, the world famous F-Plan diet. As the author of the F-Plan diet wrote, 'When people eat high-fibre diets they excrete more calories in their stools (faeces). In several experiments, scientists have undertaken the task of analysing the stools of those following high-fibre diets and have found that the calories excreted are measurably greater in number than the calories excreted by those on the normal, varied Western diets.'[7]

While there is some logic behind high-fibre dieting, taking laxatives is almost certainly a harmful waste of time. To understand why requires a brief explanation of the workings of the digestive system.

When food is eaten, it is initially mixed with saliva, chewed into soft lumps, and swallowed down the oesophagus. It then enters the stomach where it mixes with the acidic gastric juices, which break it down further. Here it is churned into a smooth paste. After passing through the stomach the food enters the small intestine, where it is again mixed with juices which break it down into digestible parts small enough to pass through the wall of the intestine. Any indigestible residue is moved by muscular waves into the large intestine, or colon. Here water and salts are extracted, and the remaining indigestible and useless residue passes on to the rectum, where it stays until it is expelled through the anus.

When laxatives are taken these tend to work by stimulating the colon – the large intestine. This will result in the bulky residue being moved on more quickly to the rectum. However, as the absorption of calories from the food will have already taken place in the small intestine, this is too late to have any really beneficial effect on weight control. They do, however, give the bulimic patient the sensation that the bowel has been cleansed – an important psychological sensation. In addition they will help to prevent the feeling of abdominal distension and bloating which follows a binge.

There are three main groups of laxative drugs which are often abused.

Bulk purgatives

These work by increasing the volume of the bowel contents, and by making the faeces less sticky. In medical practice the most useful are known as *hydrophilic colloids*, and act by holding water in the bowel, rather than allowing it to be re-absorbed. Typical examples are Fybogel, Isogel, Normacol, Bran, and methylcellulose or fibre granules. (Most of these can be obtained without a prescription.) Incidentally, some people try and use methylcellulose granules or fibre granules or tablets to help in weight control, rather than for their laxative effects. The theory is that taking them with water before a meal is supposed to create a feeling of fullness which puts the patient off their food. It is an interesting theory – but it does not work.

Faecal softeners

Rarely used by bulimics, these are mainly prescribed or recommended by doctors to avoid straining – for instance, after surgery. Typical examples are liquid paraffin, which is undigested and supposed to be a lubricant, and docusate sodium (Dioctyl) which acts by allowing penetration of water and fats into hard, dry faeces.

Stimulant laxatives

This is the group of drugs most used by people with bulimia. They increase the muscular activity of the bowel, squeezing its contents, and hurrying the bowel contents along. Too high a dose can cause abdominal cramps, and prolonged use leads to the bowel becoming resistant to their action so that larger and larger doses are needed to have an effect.

Examples of stimulant laxatives include senna (Senokot),

cascara, castor oil, Co-Danthramer, sodium picosulphate (Laxoberal), and bisacodyl (Dulcolax).

Jenny, a nursery nurse, told me about her laxative abuse. Her bingeing made her feel:

> so totally out of control when I eat. I feel bad and wicked. As I eat I find the hate for myself and the lack of control grows and grows, and the depression floods in. When I eat I always try to cleanse myself and get rid of the fat by vomiting. I will also take large amounts of laxatives. Each time I put the number up by one or two. I'm due to take 197 senna tablets tomorrow. Then 198 or 199 and so on. It costs me a bomb and my husband would have a fit if he knew. I hate to think at times what state my colon, liver and kidneys are in, but I just *have* to take them come what may. They rule my life as I plan my days around them.

Many bulimics to whom I have spoken said that they used up to two hundred laxatives each day. The average sufferer will use far fewer than this, but however many you might use, they are all useless in weight reduction – and often worse than useless. Indeed, as many laxatives also cause fluid retention, and as retained fluid causes swelling of the ankles and wrists, and weight gain, the effect can be harmful. If they were effective and helpful, then no one would feel like Kathryn:

> In 1990 I decided consciously to lose weight. I joined Weight Watchers and weighed in at fourteen stone ten pounds. I was shocked and terrified. I did follow the eating plan for the first few months, and I then became involved in the laxative and vomiting cycle. I managed to reduce my weight to ten stone, but nevertheless I still feel grossly fat, ugly, and deeply wish I could be thin. Everything I eat haunts me with the voice of 'You'll get fatter if you eat that.' At the age of thirty I am entangled in the painful circle of starvation, bingeing, and then purging. It's like being in a whirl-pool that is sucking you deeper and deeper.

Not everyone who uses purging as a method of weight control turns to medication; some try a high-fibre diet.

Christine described her morning like this:

> From the moment I get up in the morning I am
> obsessed with food. Whereas other people would
> just sit down for breakfast without giving it a second
> thought, I must eat something which will make me go
> to the toilet – i.e., a laxative type of food. If I am not
> able to excrete I panic, and I start my day very tense.
> I have seen myself not go to work because I work
> myself into such a state if I'm constipated. I think
> that I cannot function properly if I don't go every
> morning after breakfast. It is the first thing that I think
> about in the morning. Most people would get dressed
> and organised before thinking about sitting down to
> breakfast. Not me, I'm out of bed and straight to the
> kitchen. I must eat something which will make me
> go. The rest of my day is dominated by food; what
> unfattening thing I am going to have for my lunch,
> what I can eat for dinner that will be satisfying without
> putting on weight. I cannot concentrate on anything
> else but my shortcomings, my failures, my looks, the
> reasons people won't like me, the things that people
> will think are wrong with me, and so it goes.

Diuretic Tablet Abuse

Diuretic tablets cause the kidneys to excrete more urine.
The kidneys normally work by filtering the blood, and
removing water, body salts (particularly sodium and potassium), and waste products from the bloodstream. They then
reabsorb most of the water and the salts back into the blood,
leaving the waste products to be flushed away. The effect
of most diuretics is to interfere with this reabsorption. The
amount of sodium and water taken back into the blood is
reduced, and more is lost in the urine.

If you take a diuretic, you will inevitably pass more
urine over the next few hours, and during this time you
will weigh less. You will lose the weight of the urine that
you pass. However, the moment that you take a drink, the
fluid will be back in the body, and your weight will be back
to normal.

Despite what many bulimia sufferers believe, diuretics

have no effect whatsoever on the amount of fat in the body. Their effect on weight is temporary – unless you take tablets every day. Diuretic abuse can be extremely dangerous, but despite this, it has been estimated that 40 per cent of binge eaters take significantly large quantities of diuretic tablets.

Unfortunately, as with laxative abuse, the more you use diuretics, the less effective they become. The body sets up a vicious circle of fluid loss followed by rebound fluid retention. The more you take, the more you need, and the more dangerous it all becomes. The specific hazards of diuretic abuse will be dealt with in the next chapter.

Slimming Tablets

Slimming tablets seem very tempting. A tablet that dulls the appetite and takes away the craving for food would seem very attractive to someone with bulimia. While there is a place for medication in the treatment of some long-term weight problems, on its own the standard slimming tablet is completely useless.

In the past, amphetamines were used to help suppress appetite, and these had their own complications. Modern slimming pills are still prescribed by some doctors, particularly in private slimming clinics, but this still does not mean that they are safe or a sensible way to tackle weight and appetite problems. Indeed, such is the concern about these drugs that the British General Medical Council has advised doctors in the UK against using such drugs, and the *British National Formulary* (the guide to medication that is used by all Britain's doctors) states quite clearly that 'Centrally acting appetite suppressants are of no real value in the treatment of obesity since they do not improve the long-term outlook. They are sympathomimetics and most have a pronounced stimulant effect on the central nervous system.' This stimulant effect causes agitation, sleeplessness or depression.

The problems with these drugs are manifold. Except in very exceptional cases, slimming tablets like these are of no use. Despite this, like every doctor, I have patients who still go to private clinics and buy these drugs. The more commonly used names of the drugs mentioned above are Tenuate Dospan, Apisate, Teronac and Duromine. If have purchased them, my advice to you would be to flush them down the toilet. Few drugs have been more clearly condemned by the authorities who control and advise on the use of medication. They can be addictive, they can cause even more emotional and nervous upsets, and in the long run they don't work. Haven't people with bulimia got enough problems without using slimming tablets as well?

The Dangers of Bulimia

It is generally accepted that almost every type of medical problem can be considered in physical, psychological and social terms. Indeed, junior doctors in training are now taught that this is one of the cornerstones of the essential art of diagnosis.[1] Not only should one consider the physical effects of a problem – the traditional area of medical interest – but also the ways in which this is affected by psychological and social implications, and also the way in which the physical can affect the psyche. There is no such thing as a purely physical or purely emotional problem.

Even something as simple as the common cold has the potential to affect the individual in different ways. How much you suffer from the symptoms can be affected by your general sense of psychological well being. On a very simple level, the same level of cold virus will produce very different symptoms in someone who is bubbling with joy and enthusiasm than in someone who is bored with their life, tired and unhappy. And nowhere is this trinity of the physical, psychological and social more evident than in the problem of bulimia nervosa.

Not only do bingeing and self-induced vomiting very obviously have important physical effects on the body, but the loneliness, secrecy, guilt and despair all take an equal psychological and social toll. Obviously the extent to which someone suffers depends on a number of factors, in particular the length of time they have had bulimia, and how often they binge and/or purge. In addition, if they eat sensibly and healthily between the bingeing sessions then the overall effect on the body may well be diminished, compared to someone whose diet consists almost totally of 'junk' foods.

Much of this book is concerned with the psychological and social effects of bulimia, but the condition also carries a number of purely physical risks – and this chapter will take a closer look at these. The most logical way of examining the physical dangers is by looking at each part of the gastro-intestinal tract in turn. Indeed, almost every part of the gut, from the mouth to the anus, can be affected.

The Teeth and Gums

As many bulimics binge on sugary foods, there is a real risk that they will develop tooth decay and gum disease. However, there is an even bigger and more common problem. Repeated vomiting means that stomach, or gastric, acid enters the mouth. The gastric juice, which is designed to help break down and digest food, contains many chemicals, one of which is hydrochloric acid. You can imagine the effect that a mouthful of hydrochloric acid can have on the enamel of the teeth. This damage is particularly obvious on the inner surface of the teeth, and the teeth frequently become extremely sensitive to hot and cold foods. In addition, if there are fillings in the teeth, these gradually begin to protrude. The teeth become worn down, while the fillings do not.

What makes this damage even worse is that many bulimics brush their teeth vigorously after vomiting to disguise and eliminate the smell of vomit. Brushing after the teeth have been coated with acid means that the enamel can be badly scoured and this damage will be permanent. Using a mouthwash following bulimic vomiting would be better for the teeth.

The damage to tooth enamel means that many people with bulimia eventually need to have their teeth crowned, although the problem will obviously keep recurring as long as the vomiting persists. Dentists are becoming increasingly aware of the problem of bulimia and may be the first people to raise the issue with a sufferer.

The Salivary Glands

It is very common for the salivary glands to become swollen in a bulimic. These are the glands which produce the saliva necessary to help chew food, and bingeing causes them to work overtime. There are three pairs of salivary glands. The *parotid* glands lie over the angle of the jaw on each side, just below and in front of the ears. The *sublingual* glands are found in the floor of the mouth, where they form a low ridge on each side of the frenulum – the thin band of tissue that attaches the under-surface of the tongue to the floor of the mouth. Finally the *submandibular* glands lie towards the back of the mouth close to the sides of the jaw. Each of these glands consists of thousands of saliva-secreting sacs and tiny ducts carry the saliva into the mouth.

Any of these glands, but particularly the parotid glands, may become swollen. A swollen parotid gland gives a person the chipmunk-like appearance of mumps.

The Throat

Most bulimics who control their weight by vomiting make themselves vomit by pushing something down the back of the throat, whether it is a spoon handle, finger, or similar object. If much force has to be used, and it can be extremely difficult to make yourself vomit in this way in the early stages, the back of the throat may be damaged. If severe enough this can cause bleeding. Acid from the stomach can also make the throat very sore.

Nicola described her experiences of self-induced vomiting and the problems that can result:

> During my first two years at college, the chief thing that I remember is the secrecy. I would hide myself in

my room, spending hours eating anything and everything, and then sticking a spoon or toothbrush down my throat to make myself feel clean again. And then, one summer, I swallowed a spoon while trying to make myself sick. I was mortified and wouldn't admit to anyone how I'd swallowed it – I couldn't come up with a consistent reason, but I wouldn't admit the truth. I had to spend two weeks in hospital, having the spoon removed by a laparotomy. Of course they knew how I'd swallowed the spoon, and questioned me about it repeatedly, but I wouldn't own up. I couldn't own up.

In addition, some bulimics become hoarse, and can have an increased number of throat infections.

The Oesophagus

Many people with bulimia report that when they vomit they notice some blood mixed in the vomit. This may come from the back of the throat, but very rarely the oesophagus itself can tear. There have even been occasional case reports of a complete rupture of the oesophagus – a condition which requires urgent medical treatment.

On a much milder level, repeated deliberate vomiting can lead to the development of a hiatus hernia. This is a weakness of the sphincter (a muscular type of valve) at the junction between the oesophagus and the stomach. If severe this can cause repeated regurgitation of food from the stomach up into the mouth. Even a mild hiatus hernia can cause heartburn. The lining of the stomach is designed to tolerate acid, but the lining of the oesophagus is not. If the sphincter between the two is damaged, acid can get into the oesophagus, irritate the lining, and cause indigestion, flatulence and very painful heartburn.

The Abdomen

Maggie, a bulimia sufferer aged 22, wrote in a letter:

After I'd eaten I always felt awful. My stomach felt

and looked enormous. I thought I would explode.
It was no wonder that I had to clear myself out.
All that food . . . I had to get rid of it somewhere.
I simply couldn't stand it, but I simply couldn't
stop.

Bingeing obviously makes the sufferer feel bloated and
full. It is hardly surprising that abdominal pain commonly
occurs. Disturbance of the pattern of bowel motions, with
either constipation or diarrhoea, is also a frequent development after bingeing.

Laxative abuse can cause spasm of the bowel, which can
be enormously painful, and vomiting can itself cause upper
abdominal pain. Long-term laxative abuse is also likely to
cause a loss of bowel tone. This means that the muscles of
the intestine become flabby, which leads to constipation,
and even greater laxative abuse.

Incidentally, when bulimia sufferers stop using laxatives or vomiting to control their weight, they often feel
bloated and full to begin with. These have been described
as withdrawal symptoms, but they rarely last for more than
ten days. As a normal eating pattern is re-introduced the
bowel gradually recovers, but this can take time. It can
lead to an increased temptation to begin purging again,
but it really is worth hanging on. The discomfort will
pass.

The Anus

Regular laxative use can cause quite severe soreness or
itching around the anus. This is caused by passing motions
which are looser than usual, making anal hygiene extremely difficult to achieve.

The Skin

Many bulimics have very dry skin, which probably results
from dehydration. This loss of water from the body may be
caused by abuse of diuretic tablets, repeated vomiting or
excessive use of laxatives. Some sufferers find that their

fingers and toes can feel numb, and loss of hair is very common to bulimics.

The Eyes

Many bulimics have bloodshot eyes after an episode of vomiting. While this does not cause any long-term damage, it is a very visible sign of the problem. One bulimic wrote, 'After a while, I began to notice some of the little telltale signs on my face. My eyelids were swollen, and around my eyes I noticed little broken blood vessels.' Along with recurrent mouth ulcers and swollen glands, red eyes can be one of the earliest physical signs of the problem.

Electrolytes

The various salts in the body fluids are known as electrolytes and the most important of these are sodium and potassium. Anything which upsets the correct balance between them can cause major problems in the functions of the body.

Obviously, drinking enormous quantities of fluid to wash out the stomach, repeated vomiting, use of laxatives, and so on, can all severely disturb the balance of these electrolytes, leading in particular to low levels of sodium and potassium. Almost half of all bulimics show some disturbance of their electrolytes. If severe, this can have very serious effects. For instance, the normal regular beating of the heart can be affected by a fall in the level of potassium in the blood. Too little potassium can cause an irregular heartbeat. The combination of regular vomiting and laxative abuse seems to be most likely to trigger off electrolyte disturbance. These do, however, revert back to normal as soon as the bulimia stops.

Some sufferers from bulimia who are aware of the problems of electrolyte disturbance from laxative abuse try to counteract this by eating foods that contain plenty of potassium, like bananas and oranges. However, as I discussed in Chapter 4, laxative use is entirely ineffectual in controlling weight.

A low level of potassium in the blood can not only affect the regularity of the heartbeat, but can also be associated with numbness and pins and needles in the limbs, muscular weakness, low blood pressure, kidney damage and even epileptic fits.

The Heart and Circulation

Recent research has suggested that changes in the cardiovascular system are fairly common in sufferers from bulimia.[2] It is common for the electrocardiogram test (ECG) to show changes, and heart rate, blood pressure and oxygen consumption in response to exercise are all reduced.

Most of these changes result from electrolyte disturbances which are the result of repeated vomiting. The use of the drug *ipecacuanha* to induce vomiting can also have a directly damaging effect on the heart muscle.

Other Dangers of Bulimia

Oedema

Oedema is the medical term for the puffiness or swelling that can occur as a result of fluid retention. In bulimia this is very often the consequence of dehydration that results from either vomiting or laxative and diuretic abuse. The swelling consists purely of excess fluid, but it can make the sufferer feel both heavy and fat, so triggering off another bulimic attack.

In addition, there is evidence that sufferers from bulimia are more prone to both urine infections and to renal (kidney) failure.

Hypoglycaemia

Normally, when we eat carbohydrates, the body responds

by increasing the production of insulin by the pancreas. Insulin is a hormone which promotes the absorption of glucose (sugars from the carbohydrate) into the liver and also into the muscle cells, where it is converted into energy. Insulin therefore helps to prevent a build-up in blood glucose. Diabetics have insufficient insulin, which leads to high levels of glucose in the blood.

The opposite can sometimes happen to bulimics. As the bulimic eats carbohydrate-rich foods, the body responds by pumping out more insulin. But if the food is then vomited before the insulin can go to work, there is excess insulin in the body. This can reduce the level of glucose that is already in the blood, producing the condition of hypoglycaemia, otherwise known as low blood sugar.

Hypoglycaemia can cause a number of physical problems, as many parts of the body, in particular the brain, depend on an adequate level of blood glucose to function normally. Problems from hypoglycaemia can include:

- sweating;
- palpitations;
- weakness;
- hunger;
- headaches;
- double vision;
- dizziness; and
- irrational behaviour, and even feelings of panic and confusion.

It must be said that while some researchers have shown that normal secretion of insulin does not occur in bulimia sufferers who are given a test meal, others have found no differences at all. The debate as to what happens to the insulin response, and why it happens, will continue for some time yet.[3,4]

Menstrual disturbance

It has been estimated that approximately 40 per cent of female sufferers from bulimia will suffer from irregular periods, and in about one in five the periods can stop altogether. These changes can be caused either by stress, or possibly by some of the physiological changes that occur in this condition. In particular, the combination of a low body weight and a diet low in carbohydrates, can significantly affect the levels of hormones that control menstruation. It has been shown that regular menstruation depends on the body having a normal proportion of fat – usually about 20 per cent – and women with bulimia have often reduced their body fat to under 10 per cent. Inevitably this alteration of the menstrual cycle may have long-term effects on fertility. Oestrogen is fat soluble, and the human female body does require a certain amount of body fat in order to function normally. It seems ironic that skinny fashion models, who attempt to portray the ultimate in sexiness, are actually promoting a body shape that can damage normal sexual functioning. Fat is not always a bad thing.

Metabolism

Everyone is aware that there are some seemingly lucky people who can eat a great amount without ever seeming to put on weight, while others need to watch every calorie. This is not simply because life is unfair, but because different people can have very different metabolisms. The lower your metabolic rate, the greater your potential to become obese.[5]

Various factors can alter the metabolic rate, and one of the most important of these to the bulimic is low levels of food consumption. When little food is taken in, the body believes that food is scarce, and therefore conserves energy by slowing the metabolism. For instance, in one study of obese women who took a very low calorie diet (300 calories per day) their metabolism slowed by an average of 22 per cent.[6] This is a vital and life-saving defence mechanism undertaken by our bodies. In bulimia, and indeed in regular dieters, it is counter-productive to cut down to a very low calorie consumption. In other words, dieting can slow the metabolic rate, making the dieter need even less food than before. In the bulimic, who often alternates bingeing and dieting, the metabolic rate can be similarly reduced. After all, if food is vomited after a binge, the body treats this as if no food has been eaten.

The good news is that there is evidence that the metabolism can be stimulated by exercise, so that the continual cycle of dieting leading to an ever lower metabolic rate can be interrupted.[7] However, the body will only settle down to a normal metabolic rate, with no fluctuations, when the problem of bingeing, dieting and purging has been tackled once and for all.

The Dangers of Slimming Tablets

A number of bulimia sufferers do try so-called slimming tablets to help them gain control over their appetite and weight. In the last chapter I discussed why these are unlikely to help, and here will discuss how they may cause significant problems.

For many years amphetamines were used as slimming tablets. These should no longer be prescribed by reputable doctors for this purpose, and the prescription of amphetamines is now controlled by the Misuse of Drugs Act. The *British National Formulary* has stated that there is no place for amphetamines in the treatment of obesity, and has warned of the real risks of addiction and psychological problems. However, amphetamines are still very widely available as street drugs.

Amphetamines work by stimulating the secretion of chemicals known as neuro-transmitters. These are chemicals secreted by nerve endings, and they increase nerve activity in the brain, making the taker seem more wakeful and alert.

However this feeling is only present at the start. When any stimulant effect has worn off, most users feel depressed, hung-over and lethargic. This frequently leads to the desire to take another dose, and a cycle of dependency may be born. Side-effects include tremors, sweating, severe anxiety, palpitations and difficulty sleeping. In addition, hallucinations, hypertension (high blood pressure), and even fits can develop. It is little wonder that these drugs are no longer used for eating disorders.

Other appetite-suppressant drugs do exist and are used by some sufferers to control binge eating. Not only are they not successful, but they too create very significant problems. The side-effects of these drugs can be briefly summarised as follows.

Amphetamine-like drugs
These include diethylpropion hydrochloride (Tenuate Dospan, Apisate), mazindol (Teronac) and phentermine (Duromine and Ionamin). While not having all the disadvantages of the amphetamines themselves, this group of drugs can cause problems. Side-effects include a dry mouth, insomnia, headaches, rashes, increased nervousness, depression, psychosis, hallucinations, hypertension and constipation.

Fenfluramine
Although fenfluramine (Ponderax) is also related to the amphetamine family of drugs, in normal doses it tends to have a sedative rather than a stimulant effect. Despite this, it can be abused and sudden withdrawal can cause quite severe depression. Side-effects include diarrhoea, drowsiness, dizziness, and most of the other problems listed above for amphetamines.

Dexfenfluramine
This drug, marketed as Adifax, is related to fenfluramine, and appears to have significantly fewer side-effects. However, it cannot be recommended for sufferers from bulimia. In particular, it is specifically contra-indicated for anyone with a history of anorexia nervosa, psychiatric illness, depression, or drug or alcohol abuse.

Alcohol

Finally, alcohol may be abused by bulimics in an attempt to blur reality. Unfortunately, as the alcohol wears off, and regular life resumes, more and more alcohol may be necessary to achieve the same effects. The problems of alcohol abuse are really too well known to be listed in detail here. Suffice it to say that as well as physical problems such as gastritis, ulcers, cirrhosis of the liver, dehydration, pancreatitis, epilepsy and amnesia, there are also serious social problems. These include aggression, mood swings, neglect, depression, accidents, driving offences and more. If you feel that alcohol has become a problem for you, do please talk to someone about it. Your doctor would be a good person to start with. Alternatively, alcohol advice centres are available in most areas; look in your phone book. Don't ignore it – alcohol problems rarely go away by themselves.

Finally, don't forget the many emotional and social side-effects of bulimia itself. I have covered these in depth elsewhere in the book, but it is worth repeating that a condition that may cause deception, guilt, lying, and excessive spending is not likely to help inter-personal relationships and self-esteem. The physical side-effects are bad enough. Destroyed relationships can be the very last straw. Bulimia is a lonely condition and the implications of alienating the people whom you love, and who love you, are very frightening.

You need to know the problems that can be associated with bulimia, but you also need to know that the condition can be helped. The last section of this book will show you that a great deal can be done for bulimia and for bulimics. You need to be realistic, but you do not need to despair.

How Common is Bulimia?

How many people suffer from bulimia? You may have just come to terms with the fact that you, or a friend or family member, has the condition. You are bound to want to know whether this is unusual, and you'll be interested in finding out how many people share your difficulties. You may be wondering why newspapers and magazines are so full of articles on this problem? Is it really common, or does it just make fascinating reading? Indeed, is bulimia a new problem, or has it been around for years?

Unfortunately, none of the answers to these questions is as straightforward as you might like. As we have seen, the first written report on bulimia appeared as recently as 1979.[1] Does this mean that it simply didn't exist until the 1970s, or is it simply that no one recognised it, diagnosed it, or admitted to it? It is also clear that the public is becoming increasingly aware of the problem. Does this mean that the condition itself is becoming more common?

For a start, doctors only diagnose diseases that they recognise. If someone presents a pattern of symptoms that does not add up to any known disease syndrome, then the symptoms may be ignored. A classic example of this is the syndrome of Temporal Arteritis. The symptoms include headache with tenderness of the scalp, which is associated with aching in the shoulders and thighs. This condition is now recognised quite regularly by doctors, but only a few years ago it was unheard of. Does this mean that patients did not suffer from it? Obviously not. They would have mentioned this curious combination of symptoms to their doctor, and the doctor would not have recognised them as being one illness. The fact that the condition is now known to be relatively common does not mean that more people are suffering. It simply means that doctors have become much more aware of it.

And so it could be with bulimia. It is possible that bulimia may have been in existence for hundreds of years, but has only recently been recognised and named. Susie Orbach, in her book *Hunger Strike* notes that the first groups that she ran in 1972 for compulsive eaters included women who were bingeing and vomiting or else using purgatives in large quantities.[2] The condition might not have had a name then, but it did exist.

As we will see later, in Chapter 7, there are reasons why present-day pressures may have made bulimia more common, but no one can be absolutely certain. If you don't recognise something, you simply cannot confirm its existence. In addition, we have already seen that most sufferers from bulimia look normal. They are not obviously skinny, like people with anorexia. Their problem is a secret.

Incidentally, while bulimia has only been officially recognised as a medical problem since 1979, during the Roman Empire people frequently used to vomit after feasts. The Romans were notorious for their lengthy banquets, and they would eat and eat until they were absolutely full. They then retired to the special *vomitoria* where they would bring up what they had eaten, to make room for the next course. Almost certainly this was not true bulimia. It was probably simple greed. The rugby player who drinks ten pints of beer, followed by an Indian meal of Vindaloo and chips, and who then vomits on his drunken way home is closer to the Romans than to the typical current-day bulimic.

Working out the exact incidence of the disorder is more complex still. If a doctor or psychologist has an interest in a problem then he or she is likely to ask about it. Patients are more likely to tell more to someone who asks than to someone who doesn't. Those who are interested will discover more cases than those who are not.

Since I began to write this book, I have inevitably become much more likely to ask about binge eating, self-induced vomiting and laxative abuse. In my small rural general practice, I have been genuinely surprised by the very considerable number of people who have admitted to the problem. When discussing this recently with a group of doctors, I found that most had very few, if any, patients with bulimia. As they would be the first to acknowledge, they must have had exactly the same number of bulimic patients as I do, but may not have found out about them. And the chances are that a family doctor with a special interest will only know about a small proportion of cases on his or her list. Such complications make estimating the actual incidence of the problem in the overall population difficult.

Almost all studies of the condition are likely to be biased in some way. Like sufferers from anorexia nervosa, the great majority of bulimics appear to be young adults. Most people are aware of this fact, and most studies on prevalence are based on those people who seek help for the condition. However, it is possible that the age of the sufferer is instrumental in deciding whether she will seek help. If young adults are more likely to acknowledge their bulimia to doctors, then all the reports are likely to over-represent young adults. It could be that sixty-year-olds suffer, too, but never seek help, so no one knows about them.

I believe that this is a curious but important argument. The study and understanding of bulimia is in its relative infancy, and I hope that both professionals and sufferers will retain an open mind about the currently known 'facts'. Facts can only change when someone challenges them. If you are male, or middle-aged, or even elderly and are worried that the descriptions of bulimia in this book do not fit you, then remember that only you are the expert on you. You can still seek help, and you can help to educate the experts.

There have, nevertheless, been some extremely important

and helpful studies into the incidence of bulimia. However, even these are hampered by the fact that, as we have already seen, bulimics tend to feel guilty about the condition, and to keep it as a closely guarded secret. The actual incidence could be even higher than the published figures.

Many studies have examined the incidence of bulimia in students in colleges and universities. For instance, two highly detailed studies of two different female college populations in 1984 revealed rates ranging from 3.9 per cent to 18.6 per cent.[3,4] A review in 1990 of the scientific literature on bulimia suggests that the prevalence among adolescent and young adult women is probably about 1 per cent.[5] An important question is whether bulimia is genuinely becoming more common. Two studies have compared groups of schoolgirls in 1981 and 1986,[6] and also college freshmen in 1980 and 1983.[7] One said that bulimia was becoming more common, and the other said it was less common. As both studies simply relied on self-reported questionnaires, not too much weight can be placed on their findings. The case remains unproven.

Of all the many different papers that I have consulted, it appears that between 1 and 19 per cent of females suffer from bulimia. The problem in males does appear to be significantly different, and I will return to it in Chapter 14. Briefly, however, it has been estimated that bulimia affects approximately two in every thousand adolescent boys and young adult men, and that there is one male bulimia sufferer for every ten females.[8]

Why is there this apparently extraordinary difference in the results of these various studies? This is partly to do with the method – the result is going to be influenced by the way in which the subjects are recruited, whether student studies include undergraduates and postgraduates, and they obviously depend very greatly on the actual criteria which are used.

It would probably be a reasonable, educated guess, based on all the various studies, that the actual incidence is between 1 and 3 per cent of all adolescent girls and young adult women. However, this could well be only the tip of the iceberg. Several researchers have not only looked at bulimia, but have also studied the prevalence of so-called 'sub-clinical' eating disorders. This includes those whose eating is abnormal and may be characterised by excessive dieting, laxative abuse, or binge eating, but not to a level that would constitute true bulimia. In one 1989 study an incredible 43.4 per cent of female college students had a history of binge eating, and 12.2 per cent sometimes used laxatives to help control their weight.[9] A 1991 study showed that 49 per cent of females studied engaged in binge eating,[10] and an earlier publication in 1982 had showed that one in three female American college students binged, and one in eight vomited food.[11]

You only have to look at the display of slimming magazines in an average newsagent's shop to realise that dieting and weight control are big business – a topic that I will return to later – but it is still a distressing statistic to find that in a 1990 study of female college students more than one in ten were pathologically preoccupied with their weight.[12]

Who Gets Bulimia?

For some time it has been thought that bulimia nervosa and other eating disorders are much more common in people from the higher socio-economic groups. However, this may be a classic example of the truisim that you find things where you look for them. If that group is the one that has been most studied – and a majority of studies have looked at students – then of course it is obvious that the highest *recognised* incidence has been in that population.

However, recent research suggests that this may not be the case, at least in America. One particular study found no difference in eating disorders or attitudes in different socio-economic groups. Disordered eating, in all its forms, exists across every class.[13] These same researchers, however, did find that problems are more common in white Americans than black Americans. They also showed that white Americans tended to be much less satisfied with their

65

body than the black students studied. This dissatisfaction is terribly important in understanding why bulimia occurs, and is a topic I will return to in Chapter 7. Another study showed an incidence of bulimia nervosa in black American college students of 3 per cent.[14]

If certain racial groups actually do have a lower incidence of bulimia, further study of them may provide a major clue as to why bulimia occurs. If, for instance, we accept that white Western culture puts tremendous pressure on us all to be slim, and this can be shown to be a major trigger for bulimia, then the study of cultures with other beliefs may show them to have a much healthier attitude to their bodies. Perhaps white Western society may gradually change its values, but with a multi-million-pound slimming industry pushing its products on street corners, and in countless magazines, it's unlikely.

In Chapter 9 I will consider some of the social factors that might drive people towards bulimia. However, it is quite clear that any particular sub-section of society or occupation that favours the slim, or disadvantages the overweight, is going to put pressure on people to become slim, whatever the cost. And that's an open invitation to eating disorders.

It has been shown that the incidence of eating disorders in models, dancers and some athletes is significantly higher than in the general population. One study of dance and modelling students showed that 7 per cent suffered serious eating disorders. It could be suggested that people at a high risk of eating problems may be more likely to choose these particular careers. In other words, something in the personality of that person might make them more likely to become a model or dancer, and also might cause bulimia. But this is almost certainly not the case. In this particular study the majority of students with the highest incidence of problems (8 per cent) were enrolled at ten to twelve years of age, and developed their eating disorder while actively studying ballet, not beforehand.[15]

This particular study was concentrating more on anorexia, but I believe that the message can be applied to all eating disorders. In professions or courses where there is a strong pressure to be slim, eating disorders are more likely to develop. In our society as a whole, there is increasing pressure on women to be slim. Is it any wonder that the incidence of eating disorders appears to be increasing? I will return to these powerful cultural pressures, and the various theories as to why bulimia occurs, in the next chapter.

PART TWO

WHAT CAUSES BULIMIA?

7

What's Wrong with Being Fat?

Before the summer of 1981, I was a happy-go-lucky person who enjoyed life and didn't really worry about much. I had a lot of friends and was very outgoing. I mixed well and got on well with mostly everyone I met. I wasn't what you would call a stunner, but I wasn't unattractive. I had several boyfriends, but at that age I wasn't looking for anything serious. I had a very light-hearted view of life.

That summer, in August 1981, myself and my best friend went to a dance where a beauty contest was being held. During the dance, the judges asked me to go and be selected for the title. I thought that I stood no chance, and just went along for a laugh. However, to my absolute astonishment, I won. We lived in a small community, and winning really made you someone for the next year. This proved to be a turning point in my life. It completely changed my outlook, and temporarily changed my personality.

I simply didn't think I deserved the title, and I thought that everyone was of the same opinion. I thought I was too fat, and initially became anorexic. Eventually the doctor managed to get me to start eating, and that was when I developed bulimia.

Because of winning the competition I became obsessed with my looks. I started to panic about my skin, my figure, my hair. Every time I looked in the mirror I was filled up with negative thoughts: 'Look at all those spots, look how fat you are, look at your teeth' and so it would go on until I had absolutely no self-confidence whatsoever. This thought pattern along with my obsession with the way I look and my total lack of self-confidence has been with me ever since.

Obviously, few sufferers from bulimia will have developed the condition after being chosen as beauty queens, but I have quoted from Caroline's letter at some length, because she illustrates so clearly the pressures that the need for slimness can cause. But what's wrong with being fat? After all, this is the late twentieth century. Aren't personalities more important? Haven't the days of judging someone by their vital statistics passed into history?

Chapter 8 looks at many of the numerous explanations for the causes of bulimia nervosa. However, society's attitude to food and to weight are of enormous importance. The pressures and tensions that these inevitably cause are important to everyone with bulimia – whatever other underlying metabolic, psychological, environmental or other factors there might be. This chapter will attempt to unravel society's influence on women, a vital part of the problem.

Think back again to the main features of bulimia. Bulimics eat more than they need, and far more than can be explained by simple hunger. They then do anything they can to avoid the weight gain that should logically follow such binge eating.

If we lived in a society where food was just a fuel, and no one cared about our shape or size, then bulimia would not exist.

Open up almost any copy of a mainstream women's magazine. What are the articles that will almost inevitably face you? There will be recipes, or articles about food, accompanied by the most magnificent photographs. These photographs have been occasionally described as gastroporn, the stimulation and titillation of the taste buds with the unattainable. Does anyone really eat their evening meals off enormous hexagonal plates, with geometrically arranged, glistening, colour co-ordinated food? The uncollapsed soufflé of gastroporn is not the stuff of real life.

Two contrasting messages are given by magazine articles such as these, and by Western society as a whole. The first is that food is more than simple nutrition. Sharing food, preparing food, enjoying food can all be signs of love and caring. Food is fun. Food is wonderful. Temptation is there to be succumbed to.

At the same time, society also puts over a very clear message that slim is beautiful. If you want to be sexy, fit, popular, happy and successful then you have to be slim. And if you are overweight then you are probably lazy, unable to control yourself. These prejudices are learned at a very early age. An interesting study in America asked children to look at a series of six drawings of children. One was considered 'normal', one had a brace on one leg and used crutches, one was in a wheelchair, one lacked a hand, one had a significantly disfigured face, and one was fat. The children in the study were asked to rank these in order of likeability. The least liked child of all was almost always the fat child.[1]

Is it any wonder that these two messages, pulling hard in opposite directions, leave casualties? The casualties develop eating disorders, and the most classic example of all is bulimia. Other problems include obesity and anorexia. The message that slim is sexy is even frightening to anyone who is uncertain and unsure of their own sexual feelings.

Melanie may only be typical of a very small proportion of people with a weight problem, but she is certainly not unique.

> It was only after talking to a psychologist that I realised what was going on. As long as I was fat, then I had plenty of friends at college, but no one ever asked me out. I could be the life and soul of the group, but when couples paired off no one wanted me. Part of me was upset, but another part of me was relieved. The thought of sex terrified me. As long as I had my armour on, my fatness, then the boys left me alone. It was a lot easier.

Slimness and Society

Twentieth century Western society has become totally obsessed with slimness. Look at the models in advertisements, the pictures on posters, the film stars, rock stars, video stars. Look at the TV presenters, the news readers, even the female weather forecasters. They are almost all slim. Slim is successful. In 1978 a study of body types portrayed on television showed fewer than one in fifty of the actors were significantly overweight.[2]

However, it was not always so. Just look at the paintings of Rubens. The women pictured so voluptuously are hardly the waif-like supermodels of the 1990s. Indeed, they are distinctly plump. Look at paintings by Titian, or by Renoir. The women they chose to glorify in their paintings would never have had the slightest chance of being short-listed for a job in modelling in our society.

The fact is that different cultures, at different times, find different physical attributes attractive. In societies where food is scarce, and skinniness is the norm, being overweight is viewed as a sign of attractiveness and success. In societies where food is plenty, then the opposite applies. In short, whatever is the most difficult to achieve seems to be judged the most attractive and desirable.[3]

In Western Samoa, women continue to gain weight after each pregnancy until – by Western standards – they are considerably obese. However, because in Samoa fat is beautiful, they flaunt their fatness, dancing happily in a way of which few overweight Europeans would ever dream. It has been estimated that eight out of ten of the world's cultures consider a degree of overweight to be desirable for women, and in nine out of ten cultures fat thighs are deemed attractive.

Even the recent dramatic political changes in Europe have given rise to bulimia. Prior to 1989, bulimia was almost unknown in most of Eastern Europe; however, the situation is now changing. More and more cases are coming to light. Whether this is due to increasing cultural pressures to be slim, or greater honesty and openness about the illness, it is still too early to say.[4]

Look back through history. Look at the Victorian age, when women would be strapped into corsets so tight that they would sometimes faint, and even suffer broken ribs. Look at the middle ages in England, when it was considered attractive to have a protruding belly. In Renaissance Italy, plumpness was definitely in vogue, and the perfect breast size has changed not just from century to century, but within decades. Look at the voluptuous, large-breasted American 'sweater girls' of the 1950s and compare them with the slim braless women of the 1960s or 70s. Compare Jayne Mansfield or Gina Lollobrigida with Twiggy, or Brigitte Bardot and Marilyn Monroe with Jean Shrimpton. And then look at the skinny supermodels of the late 1990s.

Indeed, a fascinating academic study examining men's magazine centrefolds and the contestants in Miss America pageants, has shown a significant trend towards thinness.[5] What is particularly interesting about this study is that over the same twenty-year time span, the 'desirable' woman has become slimmer, but the actual average weight of North American young women has gone up. Incidentally, the same study also pointed out that during this time there was a significant increase in the number of articles on dieting in six major American women's magazines.

It certainly seems as if those charts which show 'Desirable weights for women' should really be re-titled as 'Weights for desirable women'. Genuine obesity is certainly a risk factor for many diseases, but the slight degrees of overweight that bother most people are simply irrelevant from a health point of view.

These dramatic swings in expected and desired sizes from year to year and generation to generation would almost make an observer from another planet think that the human body was something that you could change like changing clothes. Obviously you can't, and the dissatisfaction that this causes adds tremendously to the load of human unhappiness. No one should be surprised that people want to conform, and want to look good. It is simply that this need can get hopelessly out of control.

Dissatisfaction with one's weight and size has certainly increased in recent years. Gallup polls have shown that in 1950, 44 per cent of women believed they were overweight. In 1973 this figure had risen to 55 per cent, in 1980 it was 70 per cent, and in 1990 nearly eight out of ten of women questioned seriously thought that they were overweight.

Logically this is curious. It begs the definition of 'What is normal?' If only two out of ten women believe that they are the right weight, then does this not make them statistically abnormal?

These Gallup findings have been reproduced many times. A study in 1966 reported that between 63 per cent and 70 per cent of high school girls were dissatisfied with their bodies and wanted to lose weight.[6] A 1977 study of college students showed 75 per cent were consciously trying to limit their food intake.[7]

And there is another side to the prejudice against the overweight. Research has shown clear examples of discrimination against fat people. If you are overweight you may well suffer from discrimination in your place of work, and you are also less likely to be accepted for higher education than someone slim.[8]

Indeed, it is hardly surprising that people worry about their weight. An important and remarkable study published in the New England Journal of Medicine in September 1993 looked at the relationship between being overweight and subsequent educational attainment, marital status, household income and self-esteem in a nationally representative sample of 10,039 randomly selected young people who were between the ages of sixteen and twenty-four in 1981.[9]

Overweight in this study was defined as being above the 95th percentile for body mass index for age and sex – in other words, being in the top 5 per cent. I will define this useful measure of the body mass index on page 77.

Seven years later, when the group were followed up in 1988, the women who had been overweight (370 of the original sample) had completed fewer years at school, were less likely to be married, had lower household incomes and higher rates of household poverty than the women who had not been overweight originally. It was clear that being significantly overweight in adolescence has tremendously important social and economic consequences. The problems were greater than for those who had been asthmatic, had musculo-skeletal abnormalities, and a variety of other chronic health problems. Can it be any wonder that people become upset, distressed and obsessed about their weight?

The Slimming Business

Slimming is big business. You only need to go into a newsagent's shop to see the extraordinary number of magazines devoted to weight control, and all of them full of happy, smiling slim people, not to mention innumerable photographs of food. And it is no wonder that it is big business. It has been estimated that up to one-third of men and women in the Western world are overweight, but double this number believe themselves to be overweight. These 'normal weight dieters' can be worth a great deal of money if you are in the business. A study in Minnesota showed that only half the women who went to slimming clubs actually met any objective criteria for being overweight.[10]

In another interesting study from Canada, a questionnaire completed by a group of women showed that they believed the perfect body to be a size ten (UK size twelve). 'The perfect body is only one type, only one size. It is size ten. You may be accepted if you are smaller, but not if you are larger. To be feminine today is to be thin.'[11]

As only 8 per cent of the population are a natural size ten, this belief and pressure obviously causes very real dissatisfaction and problems. Indeed, in the UK, 47 per cent of women take a size sixteen or above. It has been estimated that in the UK approximately £25 million is spent each year on special 'diet' food and slimming aids. The book bestseller charts are regularly topped by titles such as Rosemary Conley's *Hip and Thigh Diet*,

Weight Watchers is owned by Heinz; Lean Cuisine meals are available in most supermarkets and liposuction is performed at a price by many surgeons. Other surgical procedures, from stomach-stapling to jaw-wiring are at our disposal. Helping people to reach an ideal weight is certainly big business.

So . . . What's Wrong with Being Fat?

Being very overweight is genuinely bad for your health, and likely to shorten your life. But, as we have seen, the vast majority of people who believe that they are fat are really at an entirely acceptable weight from every point of view except that of a slimness-obsessed society. Few sufferers from bulimia are significantly overweight or underweight. Indeed, bulimics frequently manage to keep their condition a total secret by the fact that their weights fall within absolutely normal parameters. In anorexia nervosa, for instance, the extreme weight loss is there for all to see. In the third type of eating disorder, compulsive overeating, the weight gain is equally obvious. But in bulimia, extreme fatness or thinness are not usually a problem.

Fear of fatness, however, is a very real problem. Why else would bulimics purge themselves with laxatives, induce vomiting, exercise excessively, and use all the other techniques for stopping their binge eating from leading to increased weight? In addition, slimming clubs – which encourage and even put pressure on people to lose weight each week – may well inadvertently encourage people to become bulimic. Imagine the scenario. You find it almost impossible to resist food. If you go back to the club, possibly with a friend, and you haven't lost weight you face public humiliation. Maybe you've been bingeing shortly before a weighing-in session. The temptation to lose weight – even temporarily – in any way that you possibly can could be intense.

So, how do you define obesity, and what is a normal and acceptable weight? Charts and tables abound. Almost every diet book contains a graph or a chart showing you what your weight should be at a given height.

Many people with bulimia are concerned, and even obsessed, about their weight. There are two main reasons why people should want to be slim. These are health and fashion. Most of the charts that are available are based on health, produced from statistics held by life insurance companies. Inevitably these figures are fairly crude. You simply cannot say that an individual's weight is an accurate guide to health or longevity. In a given individual you also have to take into account lifestyle, genetics, smoking and numerous other factors. However, weight does give some guidance and the main charts used nowadays are based on the Metropolitan Life Insurance Tables, published in 1960 and updated in 1979.[12] These tables were based on data collected from people taking out life insurance in America, and show the 'healthiest' weights for given heights in both men and women.

More recently, the Body Mass Index (BMI) has been used as a means of determining whether or not someone is obese. It sounds incredibly complicated, but it is by far the most valuable assessment. You take your weight in kilograms and divide it by the square of your height in metres. Ideally, your BMI should be between 20 and 24 for women, or 20 and 25 for men. If your BMI is between 25 and 30 you are considered to be medically overweight, and if it is above 30 then you are obese.

Let me give you an example of the mathematics involved here. Don't panic. It is all actually very straightforward if you have a pocket calculator. Let us assume you are 1.7 metres tall, and weigh 74 kilograms.

Your BMI would be:

$$\frac{74}{1.7^2} = 25.6$$

Useful, simple, relevant, and used increasingly by doctors and nurses to look at the health implications of weight.

For the vast majority of bulimics, however, these figures are also completely irrelevant. The facts of obesity cease to matter for people who are concerned with their size. The facts of fashion and attractiveness are much more important. Many people who consider themselves to be too fat have a perfectly average BMI. If this is you, then you need to ask yourself what you are too fat for. The chances are that you feel too fat to be attractive.

The role models in the advertisements or the magazines, those apparently attractive and vivacious women that so many people aspire to look like, are usually selected because they are well below the recommended lowest weight that is sensible for their height and health. It follows that countless people choose their ideal weight based on a model who is underweight, and despite being an entirely healthy, safe and sensible weight, they try to slim.[13]

In bulimia this dissatisfaction with one's shape and size gets taken to an extreme. If your self-belief and self-esteem are so totally tied in with your perception of your size, then your need to turn to the apparently extreme measures of vomiting and purging becomes all the more understandable. However, what makes this even more likely to occur is the way in which people with bulimia tend to have an entirely unrealistic view of their body size and shape.

If sufferers and non-sufferers from bulimia are both shown diagrammatic representations of women of different sizes, and are asked which figure most closely matches their own, the bulimics almost always compare themselves to the figure that is larger than they actually are. In other words, they tend to see themselves as being much fatter than they actually are. When they are asked to choose a figure which shows the size they want to be, they tend to choose a significantly slimmer figure than the non-bulimics.

Bulimics are usually unhappy on two counts. They believe themselves to be fatter than they actually are, and they want to be slimmer than is actually practical or possible. A real recipe for unhappiness.

And where do men come into all this? As bulimia is so much more a common problem in women than men, I have tended to concentrate almost exclusively on women in this chapter. The pressures on women are certainly intense. Boys and men tend to be brought up believing that society will accept them on the basis of their achievements, and how effectively they work or play. Women are often brought up believing that they will be judged on their looks. As a result of these conflicting pressures, men often become workaholics while women develop eating disorders.

However, the situation is changing. In one study in 1981 it was shown that women who are just fifteen pounds over the national average consider themselves to be fat, while men do not give themselves this label until they are thirty-five pounds above the average. It has been suggested that women believe they are fat when they think they *look* fat, whereas men do not label themselves until they *feel* fat. Things may be changing. In the past few years, naked and semi-naked male models have been used increasingly in advertising. The Chippendales, for instance, have toured, women's magazines have started to have centrefolds, and pressure may be building for men to look trimmer and to take more care of their physiques. This is something that I will be exploring further in Chapter 14.

For people with bulimia nervosa, body size and shape is of enormous significance. How much they like and value themselves is coloured almost exclusively by their feelings about their bodies. Many are desperate and even obsessed with the desire to be thin. Even the slightest weight gain is seen as a disaster. A mere pound extra on the scales can trigger off depression, and intense and excessive dieting. This then leads to rebound bingeing and the whole sad cycle continues.

And the opposite applies as well. The slightest loss of weight can cause intense happiness, totally out of proportion to the reality of the situation.

In this chapter I have tried to explore some of the facts behind society's obsession with weight, which is part of the cause for the bulimic's obsession. Perhaps when society matures and begins to judge people on attributes other than the size of the buttocks or the trimness of the waist, then much of the sadness of bulimia will become a thing of the past. But that future may be some way off. Take a look at a Barbie doll, played with by millions of small children. Barbie has a 'perfect' shape. Of course, it may simply be coincidence that more and more children are suffering from eating disorders, but if you think back to that study which showed how young children discriminate against the overweight, then it's obvious the messages that they are receiving from our society reinforce the idea that slim is in.

The immediate future is far from rosy. It has been estimated that 70 per cent of *nine-year-old* children in San Francisco are dieting because, even though their actual weight is fine, they believe themselves to be too fat. Another study from Canada has suggested that half of all six-year-old girls feel unhappy about their bodies to the extent that they are reluctant to put on a bathing costume and go to the beach.[14] There can be little doubt that a significant proportion of these children will go on to develop major eating disorders such as bulimia as they get older.

We are often shocked by some of the curious bodily distortions that other cultures have imposed on themselves: tightly bound feet in China; tribes who insert discs into the lips to make them become progressively more and more swollen and pendulous. And all the time we have a society where six-year-old girls can be self-conscious about their 'flabby' bodies. Surely we will look back on this era with amazement and embarrassment.

Physical Causes

The last chapter looked at the pressures exerted by society, but inevitably will have left you asking one vital question. Why do these pressures cause bulimia in some people but not in others? After all, we are all born into the same society. We all face the same prejudices and are exposed to the same influences. In earlier chapters I have stressed the importance of looking at the effects of bulimia in physical, psychological and social terms. The same subdivisions, familiar to countless doctors, are essential in looking at the causes.

Genetics

Is bulimia a genetic disorder? Is it something that can be inherited? Some researchers have suggested that a single genetically based biochemical disorder may be responsible for both depression and bulimia, but this is far from being completely understood. However, there does seem to be evidence that bulimia and other eating disorders can run in families. What is not certain is whether this is a genetic or an environmental link. Is your attitude to food something that is inherited, or something that you learn on your mother's knee?

Twin studies often give a clue in this type of puzzle. Identical twins share the same genes, whereas non-identical (heterozygous) twins do not. Both types of twins will be likely to face the same environmental influences. If you examine cases of twins where one twin has an eating disorder, if the twins are identical then the second twin does seem to be more likely to develop an eating problem as well. However, the studies are not yet clear-cut enough to be totally certain that environmental factors are still not the answer in these cases.

Depression

The link between depression and bulimia is both enormously complex and tremendously important. Indeed, I will be devoting an entire chapter to an attempt to unravel this topic – in particular, looking at the question of whether bulimia causes depression or depression causes bulimia. However, suffice it to say here that there can be no doubt that depression is common in families with eating disorders, and that depression can sometimes have a genetic basis. Whether being prone to depression actually increases your risk of developing bulimia or other eating disorders is not yet certain. What we can be sure of is that any link that might be proven in future will only explain a relatively small proportion of cases. Bulimia is too complex a condition to be pigeon-holed that neatly.

Biochemical theories

The last chapter examined the role of society in changing our attitudes to body size and shape, but equally fascinating is the research being done at the biochemical level. Much of this revolves around two particular chemicals – *tryptophan* and *serotonin*.

Tryptophan is one of the eight amino acids which are essential to the body. Amino acids are organic chemicals, and while most can be manufactured by the body itself, the essential amino acids have to be taken in our diets, just like vitamins and minerals.

One major line of research has examined the link between tryptophan and hunger. Many people who put themselves on a strict diet report that they feel somewhat down and depressed, and it has been shown that they also tend to have lower levels of tryptophan in their bloodstreams. After eating, particularly carbohydrates, the tryptophan level increases. This is caused by the production of insulin in response to food.

Release of insulin by the pancreas increases the blood level of tryptophan in relation to other amino acids. This raised level leads to tryptophan being passed from the blood into the brain, where it then stimulates the production of another chemical called serotonin (otherwise known as 5HT). It is the raised level of 5HT that then decreases the appetite and lifts the misery associated with it.

This isn't as complex as it sounds. To summarise the situation simply: if you have too little tryptophan in your bloodstream you feel hungry. Eating food triggers the release of insulin and this in turn increases the tryptophan level. Tryptophan then enters the brain and triggers the release of 5HT. This helps both to lift mood and to ease the hunger.

And 5HT has the potential to be one of the most fascinating chemicals within the human body. Recently, disorders of 5HT metabolism (the way our bodies process 5HT) have been implicated in a broad range of psychiatric problems. These include depression, anxiety, alcoholism, suicide, aggression and impulsiveness – all of which are more common in bulimics.[1]

I will return to the topic of tryptophan and 5HT when dealing with some of the drug treatments that are available for bulimia. In particular, it has been shown that a particular group of anti-depressant drugs, known as SSRIs (Selective Serotonin Re-uptake Inhibitors) which raise the blood levels of 5HT can have a powerful effect in many sufferers from bulimia. The best known of these is Prozac. It therefore seems highly likely that in some cases of bulimia at the very least, biochemical disturbances are of very real importance.

And what is even more fascinating is the fact that some

of the effects of diet on 5HT function appear to be specific to women. For example, among healthy women who are fed a restrictive diet for four days followed by an episode of overfeeding, changes in the ratio between tryptophan and the other large neutral amino acids were noted. It is this ratio which determines the amount of 5HT which can be synthesized in the central nervous system.[2] During the time of restricted diet it appeared that the potential for 5HT production was reduced. However, this only happened in women, and not in men. It seems as if dieting affects brain biochemistry differently in women. Could this be one of the reasons for the far greater number of women with bulimia?

Finally, the amount of a chemical, known as TRP, available in the body for the synthesis of 5HT, seems to vary with the phase of the menstrual cycle. In one study of healthy women it appeared that less TRP was available for 5HT production during the pre-menstrual phase.[3] This is, perhaps, part of the explanation for pre-menstrual binge eating – the 'munchies'.[4]

It is certainly clear that hormonal changes cause the blood sugar level to fall pre-menstrually in many women. Some women may be more aware of this, suffering cravings for sweet foods and drinks to compensate. In addition, when someone has a low blood sugar level, the body produces more adrenalin. Adrenalin has two effects. One is to lead to the release of glucose from the body stores to help correct the blood sugar level. However, as I am sure you know, adrenalin is also the chemical that is produced in times of fear, panic and tension – it's responsible for the raised heartbeat, cold sweat, dry mouth and shakiness associated with these conditions. Eating helps to reduce the adrenalin level back to normal. In other words, pre-menstrual excessive eating may genuinely help you feel better – but if you then feel guilty because of the food, a bulimic binge-purge cycle may begin again.

There can be little doubt that society's pressures to be thin do affect women far more than men. It seems possible that there are intrinsic biochemical differences between the sexes which cause this difference, leading more women than men to eating disorders like bulimia. But why should nature have made females have this curiously different way of metabolising food and controlling hunger? At the moment, there is no answer.

Secondary bulimia

Very occasionally bulimia can be a secondary problem to, or side-effect of, some other medical disorder. Diabetes and epilepsy are examples, and in certain cases the sufferer becomes wary of particular foods as he or she knows these can trigger symptoms. One way of avoiding this is bulimia. This is particularly likely to happen around puberty, a period of highly strung emotions, and subsequently bulimic symptoms may occur for emotional as well as the physical reasons.[5]

A distorted view of her weight

In the last chapter I reported the research indicating that sufferers from bulimia appear to believe they are fatter than they actually are, with a target weight and size that is significantly less than for non-bulimics. It is not yet certain whether this altered and distorted view is cause or effect. Does the distortion cause the bulimia, or does bulimia cause the distortion? Indeed, it is difficult to be certain whether it is the bingeing that causes the dieting, or the dieting that causes the bingeing.

One particularly important study that examines the way in which women with bulimia and anorexia overestimate their own body size looked at the influence of media portrayal of idealised female bodies in women's fashion magazines.[6] The authors found that if bulimic women viewed photographs of women from fashion magazines, they then showed an additional and significant increase in the estimation of their body size.

The experiment comprised twenty A4 photographs of individual women taken from fashion magazines (with the photos showing at least head down to lower thigh level), which were shown to both women with eating disorders and a group of women with no eating problems. Photographs of rooms from a furnishing magazine were shown to a third group.

After looking at each set of pictures, the subjects were given a pair of callipers and asked to estimate the sizes of her waist, chest and hips. This was repeated after the second set of pictures.

After exposure to the fashion photographs the women with eating disorders estimated their size as being 25 per cent larger than it really was. This is a remarkable finding, and the authors are keen to avoid its being extrapolated further without scientific evidence, but it seems more than likely that constant exposure to images of slim and fashionable women is detrimental to the self-image of the bulimic. They do, however, advise women with eating disorders to avoid publications which portray women in this way.

The possible physical causes of bulimia are still a long way from being fully understood; however, a few facts are gradually emerging. There does not seem to be any obvious genetic cause for bulimia, but it does seem likely that many bulimics may have a biochemical abnormality that affects the sensation and control of hunger and eating. And while it seems clear that people with bulimia may have a disturbance of the way they judge their own body size, it is also becoming clear that this can be affected by outside influences – such as fashion. Trying to unravel all the different strands of this condition remains a problem.

Psychological Causes

As well as any individual's biological, biochemical and genetic make-up, there can be no doubt that psychological factors are also tremendously important in the causes of bulimia. What is harder to be certain about is the degree to which psychological factors are actually the cause, and to what extent they result from the eating problems.

Personality

An individual's personality is obviously the single most important factor when it comes to determining their behaviour. But what exactly do we mean by the word 'personality'? Definitions vary, but one of the most precise is the definition in the *Oxford Textbook of Psychiatry* which states that personality refers to the 'enduring qualities of an individual shown in his or her ways of behaving in a wide variety of circumstances'. In other words, it is the behavioural, attitudinal, intellectual and emotional characteristics of any individual.

In a nutshell, personality is the way in which a person relates to the world. Most of us relate to those around us in a consistent way. Some of us are shy, and some are gregarious. Some people are quiet, and others are extrovert. Every individual's personality is as unique as his or her fingerprints. We may fit into descriptive groups, but no two people are the same, and the reasons that we end up the way that we do are the result of countless different factors that affect us right through our life.

Remember Caroline, the bulimia sufferer in Chapter 7 who went to a dance and was talked into entering a beauty contest. It was a moment that changed her self-perception for ever. Or what about Jane, the air hostess in Chapter 1, who lost all her confidence when she saw herself on an airline video? If you suffer from bulimia, as you read their stories – and the others throughout this book – you may have recognised and empathised with parts of these case histories, and been puzzled about others. Sometimes you will know how they feel, and at other times you will find it hard to imagine how anyone could have the feelings that are being described.

We are all a remarkable mix of strengths and weaknesses, neuroses and delights. When you are suffering from bulimia it is all too easy to focus entirely on your faults. But every single human being has strengths and good qualities and you are no different. Later in the book I will show you how to see the good in yourself, as well as the weaknesses.

You may well have come across the phrase 'personality disorder' or 'abnormal personality'. This is typically used when someone is victimised by their own personality, or when those around them suffer from it. This definition may seem vague; it is terribly difficult to know whether people with personality traits such as recklessness, inability to make relationships, and impulsive behaviour (all of which would be used by some psychiatrists to reach a diagnosis of personality disorder) are really the result of their personality, or whether these problems are caused by sociological or even biological pressures. I have yet to see conclusive evidence that psychological or personality reasons *alone* can cause bulimia. Too many bulimics have normal personalities, and too many people with personality problems don't suffer from bulimia. Psychology alone cannot be the answer, but in combination with society's pressures, biochemical changes, and the rest of the mosaic of possible causes, psychological factors are almost certain to be very important.

Indeed, there can be no doubt that some personality types do seem to be more prone to bulimia. If you are a bulimia sufferer, you may recognise many of these in yourself – but they don't apply to everyone. There is no such thing as an identi-kit bulimia sufferer. However, the classic personality features of many bulimia sufferers can be summarised as follows:

- poor self-esteem;
- easily frustrated;
- perfectionist; and, to a lesser extent,
- indecisive.

Let's look at the importance of these one at a time.

Poor self-esteem
It now seems that in a majority of bulimics, low self-esteem appears to have been a significant problem well before the bulimia first developed. Indeed, not only is this a vitally important trait in the development of bulimia, but it probably goes a long way towards explaining why it keeps going once it has started.

By self-esteem, I simply mean that the person concerned does not like herself very much. If asked to describe herself she may well use words like useless, weak, feeble, ugly, or fat. Everything that happens to her is explained away in terms of how worthless she feels. This lack of self-esteem can cloud every waking moment.

People with low self-esteem frequently find a negative explanation for just about everything that happens to them. If something goes wrong, it is of course her fault. And if something goes right, she finds another alternative explanation. I remember one patient whose self-esteem was at an all-time low. I reminded her that she had a deeply loving husband who cared for her. 'But that's because he feels sorry for me,' she said. 'And he's pretty inadequate himself. He daren't leave me.' She was completely unable to see that he loved her for what she was, or that she was worthy of being loved. And if he did indeed love her then he too must suffer a flawed personality.

Low self-esteem is closely allied to depression. When talking to patients with depression, I frequently say, 'It just seems to me that you don't like yourself very much', at which the tears will inevitably start to flow.

It seems very likely that low self-esteem *is* a problem dating back to early childhood. In the Princess of Wales' famous speech on eating disorders she stated her belief that this is likely to be the case, and as such might well be preventable. To use her own words, 'All of us can help stop the seeds of this disease developing. As parents, teachers, family and friends, we have an obligation to care for our children. To encourage and guide, to nourish and nurture, and to listen with love to their needs in ways which clearly show our children that we value them. They in their turn will then learn how to value themselves.' This is obvious, important and true, but I must stress that if you are the parent of someone with bulimia, it does not follow that the way you brought them up is inevitably the cause of their illness. There are very many factors that come into play.

Easily frustrated
The average bulimia sufferer usually finds it incredibly hard to wait for what she wants. For example, she wants to be slim but she doesn't want to go through weeks and months of dieting. She wants to be slim today – if not sooner. She will find it difficult to tolerate discomfort. If she is bloated or feels fat after an episode of bingeing, she needs to deal with it immediately by swallowing as many laxatives as it takes.

However, these feelings regarding food often mirror the individual's attitude to life in general. Many bulimics become intensely frustrated if they can't master a new skill, or are unable to do it perfectly straight away. This is a recipe for intense frustration and dissatisfaction, but if you tie it together with the negative thinking and self-doubt that also characterises many bulimia sufferers, it's easy to see where the problems lie.

Perfectionist

Perfectionism is a very common trait in sufferers from bulimia. They may have unreasonably high expectations of themselves in almost every aspect of their lives – whether it be academic, social, or simply the way they look. Even the most intelligent of bulimic students may feel that she is not as good as her peers. Whatever work she does, she believes that it could have been better. She will compare herself unfavourably, and this ties in with the negative thinking discussed earlier. So, a female student who is generally considered to be bright, attractive and intelligent may consider herself to be slow, fat, ugly and generally incompetent. The stress that results from the difference between the way the bulimic may be seen by her friends and the way that she feels about herself can be intolerable. She will become terrified that people will find out her guilty secret, and that when they do they will see through everything else and realise just how useless she really is.

Sometimes the only way that bulimics find to ease the tremendous pressure and tension of this secrecy is by bingeing and purging. What they really need to do is to confide in someone. To be honest, and open and emotional. But many find this simply too hard, and are held back by shame and self-disgust.

Indeed, this desire to do everything perfectly and to do everything *now* can be a real hindrance when it comes to dealing with and treating the bulimia. Few bulimics ever get better instantly. Treatment can take many months. The impulsive, easily frustrated bulimic all too frequently gives up when treatment has only just started. If this has happened to you, perhaps you can recognise why this happens. Somehow you have to find the patience to persevere.

Indecisive

From an early age, many bulimics have made decisions based on what they think others expect them to do. Rather than choosing an option because it is actually what she wants, she will choose the option that she believes will please someone – usually family or friends. Indeed, this indecisiveness is an extension of the low self-esteem characterising most bulimics.

Being unable to make a decision, and being frightened of making the 'wrong' decision, can be a potent source of stress. This often results in bingeing and purging – as indecisive a way of tackling diet as it is possible to imagine.

Bulimic Beliefs

One group of American writers and researchers has shown that many people with bulimia frequently have similar thoughts, which actually have little or nothing to do with food.[1] These thoughts tend to highlight many of the personality attributes that I have described earlier. If you are bulimic, how often do you find yourself thinking these?

- *I must be approved of by everyone for everything that I do.*
  A common thought, and one that links to both the tremendous need to please people, and also perfectionism. It is also self-defeating. No one will ever please all of the people all of the time. To think this way is asking for disappointment.

- *If people really knew me, they would think I was a terrible, weak, uninteresting person.*
  A self-defeating thought and the ultimate Catch-22. 'If people like me, then they don't know me. If they don't like me, they are right.' Low self-esteem and feelings of worthlessness usually account for this.

- *If anything goes wrong, it is my fault.*
  Again, this feeling is linked to low self-esteem.

- *If things don't go as I have planned, then I am out of control.*
  This ideology can loop into a typically bulimic vicious circle. Things go wrong, as they do in everyone's life, so she believes she is out of control. And if she is out of control, she is tempted to compound the damage in order to punish herself, and is likely to binge. This striving for absolute control and perfection is always doomed to failure, whether you are bulimic or not.

- *I should be in control and competent at all times.*
  This is another common but dangerous thought linked
  to the statement above. There is nothing that says
  being in absolute control is a good thing. Control often
  leads to over-control, particularly over-control of the
  emotions. And if you control or restrict yourself too
  rigorously, then inevitably something will snap. This
  is when bingeing may occur.

It's Not All Bad

If you are bulimic you may have been reading through
these various descriptions of a bulimic personality and
recognised yourself. If you feel something approaching
despair, take heart. First of all, try to remember that the
negative way you think tends to cloud and affect your
judgement about yourself. Your view of yourself is probably
wrong.

Secondly, bulimia sufferers tend to have a number of
very positive personality attributes. They are frequently
bright, helpful, highly responsible and caring. They often
are socially aware, and many are highly sociable. Just
because you have bulimia doesn't mean that you are a
bulimic and nothing else. You have good, bad and neutral
attributes, just like everyone around you. So, start to think
of yourself as being a normal human. The bulimia will not
be with you always.

Sexual Abuse

But are the childhood influences on the development of
bulimia even more significant and worrying? In recent years
numerous articles have suggested that bulimia may well
result from sexual abuse in early childhood, and the subsequent self-loathing and low self-esteem that will almost
inevitably follow. For instance, it has been suggested that
feelings of disgust with bodily femininity triggered off by
childhood sexual abuse gets entangled with concerns about
weight and shape.

In a very important research paper published in 1992,

Harrison Pope and James Hudson reviewed the scientific literature that has a bearing on this issue.[2] They pointed out that the best way of identifying a risk factor is to do a prospective study, and that no such study has yet been performed. A prospective study is one that looks forward, rather than back. In this area a prospective study would recruit a large sample of children, document those with a history of child abuse, and then follow the entire group into adulthood to see whether the abused children were more likely to suffer from bulimia than the others, when all the other possible factors have been taken into account.

But such a study has never been performed. All of the studies that are available have been retrospective. An example of the way in which this can and has been done would be to look at a group of sufferers from bulimia and compare their childhood experiences with another group of similar adults who did not have bulimia. The groups have, of course, to be very closely matched for factors such as age, sex and social class.

After examining all the studies that have been performed the authors concluded that 'current evidence does not support the hypothesis that childhood sexual abuse is a risk factor for bulimia nervosa'. While sexual abuse did emerge as an important factor in many people with bulimia, it seemed to emerge just as often in those with other emotional or psychiatric problems, but who were not bulimic.

The authors do, however, make a number of important points. Research is still needed to determine if severe abuse, or abuse occurring at a very young age, may be a specific trigger for bulimia. They also stressed that theirs was a statistical study. For the individual who has suffered sexual abuse, it is still important that this is talked about and dealt with – whether the abused person is bulimic or not.

Perhaps what is most horrifying about this study is the finding that abuse is so distressingly common. As the authors say, 'It may be more profitable, both in therapy and in research, to direct our search towards other potential causes of bulimia nervosa and, perhaps even more urgently, towards understanding the origins of the high levels of childhood sexual abuse that apparently exist in our society as a whole.'

In another very detailed study of this topic, it was suggested that simply to put the link between sexual abuse and bulimia down to coincidence is really not adequate.[3] The authors point out that the nature of reported abuse tends to be more severe in those with eating disorders than in other women, though again they stress that this doesn't prove that the one caused the other. In this particular piece of research it was however shown that when the therapist dealing with the patient judged that abuse was part of the cause, it did seem to be associated with a greater use of vomiting as a means of controlling weight, and also that the sufferers tended to have more self-denigrating beliefs following on from the abuse.

There can be no doubt that abuse does feature very frequently in the lives of people with bulimia, and that it has devastating effects on self-esteem, but it is also clear that this is not in any way specific to bulimia. Child sexual abuse does not cause bulimia.

10

Bulimia and the Family

The last couple of chapters have dealt in detail with the intense social pressures that twentieth-century Western culture has put on women. However, pressure can come from the home. As well as these national and international factors, there are very likely to be specific and very potent demands within a family. It is important to remember, however, that every person with bulimia will have been subjected to countless different pressures and stresses, and it is quite impossible to isolate the individual specific 'cause' for any one individual.

It is common sense that the way in which any child is brought up will have an enormous influence on the way that his or her personality develops. This is particularly true and important when it comes to self-esteem, and the ability of the child to develop a really good and positive self-image. We have already seen how self-esteem can be poor in people with bulimia, and anything that damages the development of self-esteem may well be a potent factor in causing the illness.

It is clear that the way in which any family functions is bound to affect all the family members in terms of their values and attitudes regarding not just food and eating, but also body size and shape. Many families of bulimics tend to over-emphasise dieting, slimness and attractiveness. Constant comments about appearance and weight are disastrous for the frequently brittle developing confidence of adolescents.

Comments about looks may extend to others outside the family. How many young people hear their family say things like, 'Have you seen Lynda recently? Hasn't she put on weight? She's really letting herself go', or 'Look at that woman over there! What a size. She should be ashamed of herself.' Oft repeated remarks like these can begin to sow the seeds of a perceived link between attractiveness, 'goodness' and weight. You start to believe that slim is good, fat (however minimal) is bad. Someone growing up in a family over-concerned about appearance may come to believe that it is essential that she retains her slimness for fear of being rejected. This can go on to merge with the normal adolescent internal conflicts between wanting to be loved like a child and wanting to be treated as an adult.

As well as these attitudes towards food and slimness, 'bulimic families' tend to have a problem with easy and open communication. Emotions are kept bottled up. We have already seen how sufferers from bulimia tend to repress their emotions. Quite frequently this is learned behaviour.

In such families there are few open outlets for the expression of anger, happiness, sadness, fear, alarm, joy or any other emotion. While some people manage to do this without real harm to themselves, many bulimics use bingeing as a way of coping with their emotions. If they cannot reach an emotional catharsis in any other way, they can do it by bingeing.

Let me stress again that the families of bulimics are not to blame. However, I do believe that it is important for them to realise the way in which their relationships can affect the person with bulimia. If relationship problems are not tackled, the situation may not be resolved. If you understand what is going on, then you have taken the first step towards change.

It is also interesting that in families where someone suffers from bulimia, there is an increased likelihood that another family member will have an alcohol problem. The conclusion that can be drawn from this is two-fold. Perhaps this is a family which has real trouble in expressing emotion; while one turns to eating disorders the other turns to drink. Alternatively, it's possible that depression runs in the family. Perhaps a genetic predisposition towards depression is making itself apparent in different ways within the family.

Obviously, both abuse of alcohol and bulimia are examples of impulsive behaviour. It may be all too clear that the activity is potentially harmful, but the individual concerned simply finds the temptation too much to resist.

Family dynamics can, of course, be enormously complicated. It is not uncommon for the person with bulimia to become the focus for the rest of the family's anxieties and fears. Rather than tackling other family problems, especially emotional ones, the bulimia distracts everyone's attention. When the bulimia is finally tackled, other problems are quite likely to float to the surface. If family members find this too stressful to cope with, there is a risk that they may persuade the bulimic that she is not improving, or that she is not doing as well as they hoped. A focus is required to draw attention away from the real problems and they are often loath to let the bulimic off the hook. Families may not even be aware of what they are doing, but the effect can be devastating. If the bulimic's fragile self-esteem is shattered by thoughtless words from a family member who is concerned about other family problems, it may take a long time to build it up again. What is clearly essential, however, is that if difficult issues are raised as the sufferer recovers, then they should be tackled, not buried.

Finally, people with bulimia frequently want to be perfect. How often do you hear the parents of young children describe their offspring as such paragons of virtue that you know the description simply cannot be true? To be described constantly as being good and clever can be an enormous pressure for a young child and this can sometimes sow the seeds of bulimia. The child who is afraid of being less than perfect, who does not believe that she is loved, even with all her faults, may become the adolescent or adult who suppresses every unhappy emotion and projects a continuing image of controlled perfection. It is vitally important that children should be loved for what they are.

However, the parents may not be to blame for this desire for perfection. The fault is actually more likely to lie in the way in which the bulimic perceives her parents. She may believe that her parents expect her to be top in all her classes, and a success at everything she does. In reality, her parents may simply want her to be happy and to do her best, not *be* the best. The fact that someone believes that her parents demand perfection does not mean that her parents really do, but perceptions can be more powerful than facts, and once her parents realise how they are perceived, then this can help them modify their behaviour. A light-hearted comment made by her parents may be interpreted in deadly earnest by the bulimic. Asking parents to change their behaviour does not necessarily mean that the behaviour was the cause of the problem.

In the newsletter of the Eating Disorders Association, a Youth Helpline counsellor wrote of the responses that she had received in a questionnaire for young people with eating disorders. She stated, 'Every correspondent has written about the pressure that they felt from their school work and family. They were keen to please, but however hard they tried their efforts went unnoticed. What would they have found most helpful? A hug. To feel that they were loved for themselves, not their academic ability or their size.'[1] It is a powerful message.

I will return to the ways in which family and friends can help the person with bulimia in Chapter 22. However, one final point is worth making here. If you either suffer from bulimia, or are the parent, brother or sister of someone with the condition, and you are invited to join in family therapy then do remember one essential thing. Family therapy does not mean treating the family. It means treating *with* the family. Bulimia does not mean that your family is sick, but exploring the ways in which the family works can help solve the problem.

11

Triggers and Spinners

> I remember overhearing my mother talking about me.
> I was about twelve or thirteen at the time. 'She's such
> a lovely girl,' she said to our next-door neighbour, 'it
> just seems so sad that she is so chubby.' I look back on
> that as the beginning of the bulimia. That was when
> I became determined to show the world that I could
> be perfect, that I would control my eating.

It is often a chance overheard remark like this that sparks off
bulimia. Sometimes the remark is a positive one: 'Doesn't
she look lovely now she's lost weight?' Sometimes it may
be negative: a nickname, a comment, a joke. Sometimes
it may be determination to be accepted by the crowd, to
appeal to a particular boyfriend, or to avoid being teased.
The triggers need not seem to be dramatic. The results often
are.

The last three chapters have looked at some of the
causes that might begin to explain the existence of bulimia
nervosa. We have seen how bulimia does not, and probably
cannot, exist outside Western cultures which put a pre-
mium on slimness. We have seen how a complex mixture
of physical, biochemical, environmental, social, family and
other factors may predispose an individual to bulimia.

It seems likely that bulimia probably needs a combination of these in any one individual before it takes
root. We are all subjected to the same cultural pressures, but we don't all suffer from bulimia. Perhaps an

individual has to have some sensitivity, some predisposition to the condition, which then acts as a potent final trigger to bring out all the symptoms and signs of bulimia.

I have already looked at bulimia in terms of a vicious circle. Whatever the possible physical abnormalities that may predispose to the condition, it is the psychological factors which tend to keep it going. Think back to the main psychological feature of someone with bulimia – a desperate lack of self-esteem. In a society where physical attractiveness counts for so much, the bulimic will highlight what she perceives as her failings. If she has acne, every time she looks in the mirror she will see nothing but the spots. When she looks at her reflection in the mirror, or in the window of a shop that she is walking past, she won't see her good qualities – she will consider herself to look gross, ugly. Of course, other people looking at this same body may see none of this. They may see an entirely normal-looking individual. But a bulimic's vision of herself may have little contact with reality.

This perceived fatness drives the bulimic into dieting. A typical bulimic will start each day with a resolution to diet strictly, having no breakfast, the tiniest of lunches, and no snacks, with the intention of keeping the day's calorie intake below a few hundred calories. As the day goes on, the hunger gets worse and worse. The bulimic will begin to crave carbohydrates. And eventually something snaps. Dieting of this degree is very likely to lead to rebound over-eating – sometimes just of everyday foods such as crisps and biscuits. Often it simply gets out of hand.

> I just got desperate. I'd eat anything and everything. You may not believe this, but while I was living at home I would eat absolutely anything behind my parents' backs. If I was in this desperate eating mood I would even take the dog's biscuit. When he looked for it again in his box where he'd left it before dozing off, he'd snarl at his back leg as if he thought that it had

101

eaten it. Thirteen years on he still snarls sometimes at that back foot. Just think. A dog with psychological problems because of my bulimia!

As we have already seen there are many explanations for this rebound binge eating, and I will consider further theories in this chapter. In bulimia the overeating takes the form of binge eating, and as the bulimic tends not to be overweight, something has to be done about the enormous calorie intake if the condition is to be kept a secret. And the solution may be self-induced vomiting.

The vicious circle continues to go round. Because they have discovered that self-induced vomiting prevents the weight gain, the brakes are off for the bulimic. There seems to be no reason not to binge, if vomiting does away with the associated weight gain. But bingeing and vomiting do terrible things to self-esteem, and the bulimic becomes trapped in the circle. While bingeing and purging often start as an

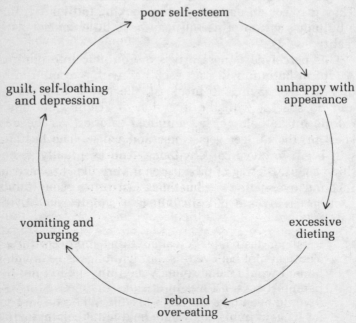

Fig. 4. The vicious circle of bulimia

attempt to lose weight, the longer the bulimic goes on, the more it becomes an important way of dealing with emotion.

I have called this chapter Triggers and Spinners because it is apparent that in any individual bulimic there can be a number of specific trigger factors that set the vicious circle turning. And once they have set the wheel in motion there are other factors, the 'spinners', which keep it turning.

Triggers

Perhaps the best way of understanding some of the personal stresses that can set up the cycle of bulimia is to look at a selection of individual case histories.

Helen's experiences were not unusual.

> As far back as I can remember I had always felt fat and frumpy. I turned to food for comfort for many years, and tried dieting on many occasions too. The 'big' diet began at the end of summer 1990 when I was thirty years old. I had no plan or target weight. I just cut back on food. A couple of months later I had lost nearly two stone. I felt good, got promoted at work, and had my first sexual experience. My world was perfect!
>
> Then the relationship ended, work became very stressful and I began to put on weight over Christmas. I began to diet again, progressively eating less and less. I began taking laxatives. If I lost weight everyone complimented me, but when Christmas came round again I suddenly lost control and put on weight yet again. I dieted and dieted and then discovered 'the answer'! I could eat all I wanted and stay the same size. To begin with it seemed marvellous, but then I realised I was bingeing every day, sometimes two or three times. At the worst it got so bad that I couldn't go for more than a couple of hours without bingeing on something. Often on the way home from work I would have to go into the public toilets to do it. I felt worse and worse. More and more disgraceful. I

felt desperate for help, but as nobody had the least idea that I had a problem it was almost impossible to come out and admit to it. I just felt awful.

It is almost certainly not a coincidence that the peak time for bulimia to start is the late teenage years. This is obviously a time of tremendous stress and major changes in one's life. This is the age of moving on from school to either higher education or work, and of breaking away from home to a newly independent life. Very many people feel quite desperate at this stage of their life, lonely and depressed. While some might turn to alcohol or drugs, others start to eat to help ease their tension. And they soon discover two things – it can be almost impossible to control their intake of food, but there is a way of controlling whether the food stays in the body.

I felt wonderful when I discovered 'the answer'. For a short while it seemed so simple. So great. And then, quite simply, I began to hate myself for what I was doing. Though, if the truth be known, I think I hated myself all along.

Spinners

The 'spinners' are the forces and feelings that keep the vicious cycle turning. Virtually every step around the cycle can become a major factor. Marion, another bulimia sufferer, describes how her self-esteem affects the way she feels.

I can't help it, but I am simply obsessed by my appearance. I can't stand people looking at me as I think that they will see every mark on my face (my skin plays up when I'm depressed) and that makes my face itch terribly. I sometimes think I'm mad. I am very sporty, but when I get depressed I become very withdrawn and make all kinds of excuses for not being as active as I usually am. This, of course, adds to my depression and I feel very down and don't want to do anything. I eat more, and start to binge, and am less active, so I put on weight which in turn gets me down, and the longer this goes on the more trapped I am in a vicious cycle. To look at me, nobody would think I was depressed, but I get to the stage where I have absolutely no self-confidence. I feel unworthy, hopeless, ugly, fat, spotty, useless and it gets to the stage where I wish I was dead.

Both hunger and dieting itself can be important spinners. The fact that you are dieting inevitably means that you think about food most of the time. As one compulsive overeater said, 'Thinking about food becomes something you do almost every waking minute. All of the energy that you could be putting into other areas of your life goes into thinking about what you will and what you will not eat.' Thinking about food without allowing yourself to eat can take the most extraordinary amount of self-control, and eventually you hit overload. A binge begins.

There have been a number of fascinating studies examining the effect of dieting on food intake. In one, a group of experimental subjects were told that they were involved in a study of how hunger affects their sense of taste. They were told that they would taste a number of snack foods and record their impressions. They would then have a second session four hours later, where again they would taste snacks and record the taste sensations. They were also told that half the group would be allowed to eat between the two sessions, and the other half would not.

The people under study were then given the first supply of snacks, and told which group they were to be in. In fact, the researchers were studying something quite different. The second session never occurred, and was not needed. What was discovered was that the group who thought they would not eat again in the four hours before the second snack test ate significantly more than the others. The very thought that they might go hungry actually made them eat more. The researcher who carried out this experiment thought that this could explain why dieters who break their diet tend to overeat. They are eating extra in anticipation of having to return to the diet.[1]

Of course, binge eating does not only occur in bulimia.

Approximately half of all overweight people have admitted to binge eating at least once per week. Dieting itself is much of the problem. Take, for instance, a box of chocolates. If you are on a diet, then you will almost certainly feel overwhelmingly tempted to eat them. It builds up in your mind to such an extent that you end up wanting and perhaps eating the whole box. If you can approach it as something that you are allowed, and simply ask yourself if you are really hungry for a chocolate or two, then the chances are that you will have just one.

Overweight binge eaters have one problem. Bulimics have quite another. Bulimic binge eaters are embarrassed, ashamed and terrified of being found out. As they also tend to be of normal weight, they also need to dispose of the enormous excess calorie intake they have consumed during a binge. And this is where purging and all the other problems begin.

Many people with bulimia have very real problems in expressing emotion. This leads to a build-up of internal stresses which can greatly worsen the situation. Take the example of Laura.

> Certainly I don't express anger or grief. I repress these feelings. The various losses I have had throughout my life I have blamed myself for. I've taken them out on myself. I don't let people see the depressed and lonely Laura. I constantly have negative thoughts about myself. These occupy my mind constantly and daily. Even when I'm doing things I can't seem to concentrate on what I'm doing. If I'm sitting down writing, I feel guilty and think that I should be doing something to help burn up more calories. I then get very depressed about it and eventually cave in on myself and shut myself away. That's when these obsessive thoughts I've had about my appearance really come into action.
>
> And as far as expressing anger goes, I simply don't show it. I take it out on myself. If someone annoys me, I don't face up to them and say what I think. I really let them get to me. People tramp all over me and I just take it. I feel like I'm being used a lot of

the time but it's my own fault. People know that I'll put up with things rather than stand against them. My current anger is with my parents, my father in particular. I need attention. I need comfort. I need help. I need sympathy. But because of dad, all attention is focused on him. Everyone thinks that I'm managing fine and just lets me get on with life as though nothing was wrong. Underneath this apparently confident and coping Laura, is the real Laura – lonely, depressed and mixed up.

No description could better illustrate so many aspects of the stresses which can keep bulimia in control. Anyone who believes that bulimia is simply a problem of vanity only has to listen to the heart-felt pleas of someone like Laura. Bulimia hurts. And bulimia is often caused by pain. People with bulimia really do deserve a great deal of understanding and help. And listen, too, to Susie.

I've had bulimia now for fifteen years, and every day is a living hell. I promise myself every night that tomorrow I will gain control again, but no tomorrow ever comes. I often wish I was an alcoholic or junkie as you can avoid coming into contact with drink and drugs. But food is different. As a mother I have to do food shopping, I have to prepare food, I have to cook food, and then my will-power gives in and I eat and eat and eat the horrible stuff. It leaves you feeling a big failure, big and unacceptable. Trapped at home, not wanting to see people any more. Just wanting to hibernate.

The importance of understanding vicious circles is that it can help you realise what is happening, and where you might be able to act to stop the wheel turning. In the final part of the book I will show you plenty of positive suggestions, but looking at the vicious circle theory you can soon see why Susie is failing. Her desperate need to gain control by stricter and stricter dieting is almost inevitably doomed to failure. The answer is to look elsewhere.

And it is important to realise that sufferers from bulimia do find many positive advantages to bingeing. Bulimia may be a way of getting rid of upsetting thoughts. It can be a way of rewarding themselves after a bad day. It can be a comfort after an emotional upset. Everyone – whether bulimic or not – uses food as a comfort. And it can also be a form of self-chastisement – 'I know I'm a useless person; I have no self-control and this proves it.' Finally, it is vital to remember that while purging may initially be only a part of weight control, it later becomes something quite different. The whole activity of bulimia develops into an infinitely more complex way of dealing with emotion. Remember this when it comes to considering how to help the bulimic.

12

Depression – Cause or Effect?

Many people with bulimia are depressed. The depression worsens their bulimia, and the bulimia worsens their depression. It is however unclear whether treating the depression makes the bulimia go away, and vice versa.

Attempting to solve these problems is an important part of understanding bulimia. It is also essential that bulimics and their families understand the whole concept of depression. Sufferers from depression, whether bulimic or not, frequently feel inadequate and guilty – as if they should be able to 'pull themselves together'. Family and friends are often puzzled, having experienced only the normal, everyday feelings of unhappiness. The term 'depression', as used by doctors, psychiatrists, and psychologists, refers to a totally different beast to the very natural unhappiness and feelings of being fed up that everyone suffers at times.

A Brief Guide to Depression

Before considering the specific role that depression may play in bulimia, it is worth examining the whole problem of depression itself. After all, feeling fed up is a nuisance. Full-blown depression can be a worrying and frightening event that can devastate those who suffer from it and all those around them.

Although there is still much debate about the topic, it is generally thought that there are two main types of depression, though with a very considerable and poorly understood overlap between them. One form, known as *reactive* depression, is a response to problems and stresses, and usually has a clearly identifiable cause. Depression that occurs following a bereavement is a typical example of this. The sufferer can be deeply and desperately unhappy, but the reason is relatively obvious and understandable.

The other form of depression is known as *biological* (or *endogenous*) depression and can occur in anyone at any time. There need not be an obvious trigger for it, and frequently the sufferer says that she has no actual worries and problems of any sort and simply cannot understand where these feelings have come from. However, it must be said that it does not only affect those without problems. It can also affect those who *are* under a great deal of stress, and these people are likely to blame their feelings on their stress.

In trying to ascertain whether someone is suffering from depression, doctors frequently use a specific checklist of questions. Accurate diagnosis is essential; without it there is little chance of offering the correct treatment.

The typical symptoms of the biological form of depression can include any or all of the following:

- poor sleep – waking early in the morning, rather than having difficulty getting to sleep;
- poor concentration;
- inability to make decisions;
- being snappy and irritable;
- loss of appetite;
- loss of interest;
- a feeling of being worthless and useless, often combined with a sense of persecution;
- lacking in energy;
- variable mood through the day, with mornings generally being worse than evenings;
- diminished or no interest in sex; and
- in addition, some people suffer other physical symptoms such as headaches, abdominal pain and constipation, as well as the very deep feeling of despondency and unhappiness that can last for several weeks, at least.

110

In contrast, patients with reactive depression often have difficulty getting off to sleep and then find it difficult to wake on time, may feel over-active and anxious, rather than drained and lifeless, and may find their symptoms worsening rather than improving as the day goes on.

This pattern of symptoms can be as obvious and meaningful to a doctor as the spots of chickenpox or the headache of migraine. Biological depression is almost certainly caused by biochemical changes in the brain, and if you find it hard to accept that minor biochemical changes can cause profound mood changes, then just talk to any woman who suffers from severe Pre-Menstrual Syndrome (PMS). Her life, finances, family and general situation remains unaltered, but her mood can swing dramatically with the phases of her menstrual cycle, purely because of influence of chemicals, such as hormones, in the blood. The brain, and the mood centre of the brain, are every bit as prone to malfunction as are teeth, kidneys or hearts.

While depression is frequently caused by biochemical changes in the brain, there is some evidence that there are certain types of people who are more likely to suffer from depression. These include:

- people who have had painful illnesses, such as back pain, for a long time – particularly if this interferes with work or other interests;
- people with another family member who suffers from depression;
- anyone suffering from a physical illness, such as flu or glandular fever, which are particularly likely to trigger an episode of depression;
- women, immediately following childbirth, although post-natal illness can strike up to two years after the event;
- people taking medication that may cause depression, particularly certain treatments for high blood pressure, steroids, and sometimes the oral contraceptive pill;
- people with a tendency to take excess alcohol; and
- some people with personalities which tend to swing from mood to mood. While we all have days when

we feel either happy or sad for no particular reason, there are people whose mood swings fairly dramatically and are said to have *cyclothymic* personalities. An excessive downswing in mood can result in an episode of depression.

It has been estimated that around one person in twenty-five will experience at least one spell of depression that is severe enough to need help from a doctor. Biological depression certainly seems to run in families, and there are particular times of life that do seem to make an individual more susceptible to a depressive illness. These are particularly adolescence, middle-age and the years after retirement.

While unhappiness that is the result of a problem in your life can sometimes be self-treated by such simple measures as giving yourself a short holiday or evening out, and by talking your problems over with a friend or counsellor, there is little doubt that the biological form of depressive illness does require medical attention. The good news is that such treatment can be extremely effective. The type of treatment that is used, anti-depressant medication, is quite specific to this problem, and such tablets are not tranquillisers, and are not addictive. The huge majority of cases of depression can be treated simply and satisfactorily by family doctors, either by medication or psychotherapy, and only occasionally do patients need to be referred to see a psychiatrist.

Depression and Bulimia

There can be little doubt that very many people with bulimia are depressed, and indeed there is a high frequency of suicide attempts and depression in patients with bulimia who are at a normal weight. One major study found that 37 per cent of the thirty bulimics in the study had made at least one previous suicide attempt,[1] while another study of seventy-four bulimics revealed that 36 per cent had attempted suicide.[2] Nothing is a more clear indicator of severe depression than attempted suicide (although – of course – not everyone who attempts suicide is clinically depressed). Depression in bulimia may be of either kind. It may be biological and biochemical, and it may run in families. There is an increased family history of depression in bulimia[3,4] and in some bulimics treatment of the bulimia may bring forward symptoms and feelings of depression that had hitherto not been apparent.

It is possible that the same form of underlying biochemical abnormality features in both depression and bulimia, a theory I have discussed earlier. However, it is also perfectly possible that having a parent with depression may be a potent cause of someone growing up with poor self-esteem, which in itself is a risk factor for bulimics.

However, depression in bulimia may also be reactive – reacting to the bulimia itself. So many bulimics feel self-disgust and guilt, feelings which themselves are likely to trigger depression. Many bulimics state that their symptoms tend to be worse when they feel depressed. There has been controversy for years about which comes first, but an interesting study from America showed that teenaged women were twice as likely to be depressed as teenaged men who were matched in every other way. The authors concluded that the women's preoccupation with their weight and body shape was the main factor that accounted for the difference.

You would think that the problem could be simply solved by finding out whether the depression happened first, or whether the initial problem was bulimia. A number of scientific studies have looked at this. In one, it was found that 59 per cent of normal-weight bulimics, and 80 per cent of anorexic bulimics had experienced major depression at some time in their lives, and among these the depression came before the eating problem on 40 per cent of occasions.[2] A very similar finding resulted from a further study, in which the depression came first in 44 per cent of the patients.[5]

However, the debate remains complex. One important review of all the published papers to date suggested that there was little or no evidence for the suggestion that bulimia is simply a form of depression.[6] The authors pointed out that many studies were flawed or biased, and they believed that bulimia and depression are clinically distinct entities. Another review has suggested that the depression is almost certainly secondary to the disturbed eating patterns.[7]

This argument is tremendously important in unravelling some of the causes of bulimia, and in helping the theoretical development of treatments, and while I do not wish to underestimate it in any way, for the individual sufferer with bulimia and depression, such debates are almost entirely academic. It's like having both a dreadful sore throat and a chest infection. The last thing you are interested in is which caused which, or whether they are linked. You just want to be able to swallow, and to stop coughing!

Coping with Depression

Bulimia and depression are so intertwined that it is also difficult to differentiate between the advice and help offered for each aspect of the problem. If you are a sufferer, tackling bulimia, using the ideas and suggestions given later in this book, will inevitably involve looking at your depressed feelings. Almost inevitably, as you begin to deal with the eating problem, you will find other feelings coming to the surface.

Whatever you do, don't hide these feelings away. Part of the reason that you have bulimia is because you cannot or will not express your feelings. You may feel that you cannot trouble other people with your worries. Why not? What is so unimportant about you? Are you sure that it isn't your poor self-esteem that is making you think others aren't interested or won't care? Remember, other people probably think more of you than you do yourself.

You may feel that it is noble to soldier on without troubling other people. Don't. Talk to someone you feel safe with. This might be a member of your family, your partner, a close friend, someone you have met through a self-help group, or a professional such as a doctor or psychologist.

Finally, you may be prescribed medication. Anti-depressant medication is not addictive. It is not a tranquilliser, like Valium. And anti-depressants are not happy pills. They do not make you artificially happy. If someone who is not clinically depressed takes them, then they will only experience the side-effects. Anti-depressants appear to act by correcting some of the underlying biochemical abnormalities that occur in depression. This is a purely physical treatment, like taking insulin to treat diabetes, or antibiotics for pneumonia.

It is absolutely essential to take the dose that is prescribed for as long as it is prescribed. Most treatment failures result from either inadequate dosages or treatments that have not been taken for long enough.[8] Many people are tempted to take a smaller dose as part of a reluctance to be on medication, and a leftover fear from all the well-publicised problems with tranquillisers. But one particular anti-depressant has been found to have specific benefits in bulimia nervosa. I will be returning to this in detail in a later chapter.

Whether or not you are given medication, your depression still needs to be tackled. Remember, suppressing your emotions may have been part of the cause of your problem. Now is the time to let them out.

PART THREE

SPECIAL CASES

13

Anorexia Nervosa and Other Eating Problems

Bulimia is obviously only one of the major eating disorders, but it is one of the most common. It is clear that there can be considerable overlap between conditions such as bulimia nervosa, anorexia nervosa and compulsive overeating. This chapter will look briefly at some of these problems, showing the important differences and similarities between these illnesses and bulimia. Some people suffer from more than one of these problems during their lives.

The very existence of the phrase 'eating problems' or 'disorders' suggests that there must be an opposite condition, that of 'normal eating'. While most people do eat normally, almost nobody eats perfectly. We all eat things that we know we shouldn't, at times we obviously shouldn't, for reasons that only we understand.

In fact, the main difference between people with eating disorders like bulimia or anorexia and so-called 'normal eaters' has a great deal to do with emotions. People with eating disorders feel out of control of their eating. They feel guilt, fear, anger, self-loathing and despair. Their pattern of disordered eating keeps on repeating itself. Most normal eaters make mistakes, learn by them, but don't get inordinately hung up about them. Life goes on, without being dominated by food, weight and feeding. For those with eating disorders, these become, overwhelmingly, the most important matters in their lives.

And one astonishing fact about the eating disorders is the almost unbelievable level of research that is currently being conducted into them. It has been calculated that the already massive scientific literature on this topic is growing at the rate of more than 100 publications per month.[1] Indeed you only have to look at the References (pages 206–215) in this book to get a flavour of the vast amount of research that is going on.

Inevitably, therefore, a summary of anorexia nervosa that lasts for only part of one chapter in one book is going to be very basic. But it is still possible, and important, to give an account of this important condition.

Anorexia Nervosa

While almost everyone has heard of anorexia nervosa, and the phrase is one that has passed into everyday language, it is still described as a 'slimming disease' – a disease caused by dieting. It is not. It is an emotional disease which focuses on food. Sufferers from anorexia have lost the ability to allow themselves to satisfy their appetite, and like bulimics they have problems living with themselves and with others. It is even possible that it is all part of the same basic disorder as bulimia, but there are real benefits in describing both conditions separately.

The word 'anorexia' simply means 'lack of appetite'. Anorexia can result from physical illness such as cancer, or even flu. It can be caused by certain medication, particularly drugs used for cancer chemotherapy and also amphetamines, and may be associated with clinical depression. However anorexia nervosa is a very different problem altogether. The term was first used as long ago as 1873 by an English doctor, Sir William Gull; although his original description was astonishingly accurate, he was wrong in choosing the word 'anorexia'. People with anorexia have a perfectly normal appetite, but however hungry they are, they suppress it. They want to be thin, excessively slim, and are frightened that when they eat they might lose control. Incidentally, while Sir William Gull was the first person to use the term 'anorexia nervosa', the first-ever description of a patient who clearly had the condition was as long ago as 1694, documented by another English physician, Dr Richard Morton.

Centuries later, the noted expert in eating disorders, Professor Hilde Bruch described anorexia nervosa as 'the relentless pursuit of thinness through self-starvation, even unto death'.[2] This tragic condition is summarised in the American Psychiatric Association's DSM-III (which we last met in Chapter 1) where it is defined as having the essential features of a fear of becoming obese, disturbance of body image, significant weight loss, refusal to maintain a minimal normal body weight and lack of menstruation (in females).

You may recall the strict DSM-III criteria for diagnosing bulimia nervosa. There are similar criteria for the diagnosis of anorexia nervosa, and these are as follows:

A   Intense fear of becoming obese, which does not diminish as weight loss progresses.
B   Disturbance of body image, e.g., claiming to 'feel fat' even when emaciated.
C   Weight loss of at least 25 per cent of original body weight or, if under eighteen years of age, weight loss from original body weight plus projected weight gain expected from growth charts may be combined to make the 25 per cent.
D   Refusal to maintain body weight over a minimal normal weight for age and height.
E   No known physical illness that would account for the weight loss.

But what does anorexia nervosa feel like? What lies behind these technical terms and the scientific criteria? Can anorexia lead to bulimia? Naomi wrote to me about her experiences.

> I had suffered from anorexia for about one year before I experienced a bulimic event. During this time I had very little knowledge of eating disorders. I really had no idea that my carefully controlled calorie intake

and excessive exercise programme was anything to do with anorexia. I felt that my preoccupation with calories and food was almost natural. After all, many of my friends seemed to be the same. We all followed similar lifestyles, glorifying in the requirement to be thin. I know that my parents disapproved, but the thought of being fat disgusted me. Nothing would make me risk putting on weight.

My first experience of a bulimic episode occurred after pressure from my parents for me to gain weight. Though I was very reluctant, I ate a meal considered normal by everyone else's standards, but for me it felt gross and wrong. I consumed in one meal my usual calorie intake for a week of 'meals'. Horrified at the thought of gaining weight, and in sheer disgust and desperation, I attempted to purge myself of the food in the only way that I considered possible – vomiting. Failing miserably to bring the food back, I turned to the next alternative – laxatives. I honestly believed that the tablets would empty my body of calories, and that I would not absorb any of the foods I had eaten.

And so it went on. Very soon I became trapped within a circle of eating foods to convince people of my normality, while also bingeing and purging to satisfy my own cravings.

When examining the various aspects of anorexia nervosa I will make an effort to point out the differences between that and bulimia nervosa. However, it is important to realise that up to half of all people who suffer from anorexia may go on to develop bulimia.

How common is anorexia?

A large recent study in South West London, looking at a population of half a million people, suggested that the incidence was one in 2800 of the total adult population or one in 1400 of the adult female population.[3] In other words it affects about one girl in every 1000 aged between 3 and 25, and so it is only about one-tenth as common as bulimia nervosa, which affects about one in a hundred at the same age. It may be becoming more common, but it is also possible that as it has become better known, so more parents will recognise the signs of the condition and seek help. Family doctors, too, are more likely to take it seriously and refer cases to specialists for help. All these changes make it difficult to be certain that it really is becoming more common, but most researchers do seem to believe that the actual prevalence has increased over the past thirty years or so,[4,5] and this is almost certainly linked with society's current cultural preference for slimness as its ideal, as discussed in Chapter 7.

Who gets anorexia nervosa?

Like bulimia, anorexia nervosa is very much more common in females than males. Indeed, it occurs about fifteen times more often in women than men, and usually begins during the teenage years. Bulimia, of course, can and does begin in teenagers, but frequently begins between the ages of twenty and thirty-five, and may even develop at any time up to the mid-forties.

Sufferers from anorexia nervosa are most likely to be middle-class, while bulimics can come from every social group. As long ago as 1880 one researcher commented that anorexia nervosa was more common in 'the wealthier classes of society than amongst those who have to procure their bread by daily labour.'[6] Anorexics also tend to be more shy and retiring, while bulimics are outgoing. Finally, anorexics tend also to be sexually inexperienced, in contrast to many – though clearly not all – bulimics.

What are the symptoms?

Almost always, the trigger that starts anorexia is a feeling that one is 'fat'. Like countless other teenaged girls, the future anorexic begins by counting calories. Unlike most of her friends, she not only sticks to the diet, but manages to reduce her calorie intake quite dramatically. Weight loss can be dramatic. Not only does she diet down to her original target level, but then far below this – usually eventually maintaining it at an average 45kg.

Food becomes an obsession. Diet is controlled with an almost superhuman rigidity, to the extent that one anorexic is reported to have said, 'I won't even lick a postage stamp – one never knows about calories.' In fact, the name anorexia is singularly inappropriate because most anorexics have retained their appetite. They are just so aware of every calorie that they resist eating as much as they can, particularly when it comes to carbohydrates.

Other anorexics use bulimic-type purging and vomiting to help their weight control even further. The average anorexic begins to look emaciated and grossly thin, in strict contrast to the typical bulimic whose weight and shape are usually perfectly normal. It is much easier to hide the fact that you have bulimia than it is to hide anorexia.

As well as losing all this weight, female anorexics often stop menstruating, or else – if they haven't yet started their periods when they develop anorexia – their menstruation is delayed. This appears to be caused by hormonal changes which are linked to the amount of fat in the body. The human female needs a certain amount of fat for normal hormonal functioning and menstruation,[7] and it is probable that this evolved to ensure that child-bearing females had sufficient spare nutrition available (in terms of reserve fat) in case food became scarce during pregnancy. A similar cessation of menstruation has been noted in marathon runners, who also lose much of their fat stores.

Indeed, people with anorexia nervosa do tend to exercise excessively, and many exercise vigorously for several hours each day. But despite this, their self-starvation, and their obviously poor nutrition, they frequently claim to feel absolutely fine, and certainly not tired. In one intriguing investigation, people with anorexia nervosa in one community were found to walk an average of 6.8 miles per day despite their emaciation and poor nutrition, while other normal-weight women in the same community were found to walk an average of 4.9 miles each day.[8] What is particularly fascinating is that in a laboratory experiment using animals, it was found that restricting food intake led to increased activity, and this in turn lead to further reductions in intake of food.[9] Could this be part of another vicious circle in keeping anorexia nervosa going?

Why does Anorexia Occur?

Anorexia nervosa is almost certain, like bulimia, to have numerous possible causes. It seems likely that there is an interaction between mounting concerns about weight and size, along with psychological and emotional problems and disease, which eventually push the sufferer, usually an adolescent, over the threshold into anorexia.[10]

In other words, society sows the seeds of an over-obsession with slimness, which then take root in someone who has either emotional or physical factors, and grows into anorexia. In people with anorexia the obsession with body weight becomes totally absorbing. There is evidence that anorexics see themselves as being heavier than they are. This has been demonstrated using a fascinating method called the 'distorting photograph technique'. This allows the subject to adjust a photograph of someone so that the image appears anywhere between 20 per cent smaller and 20 per cent bigger than the subject's actual width. Looking at photographs of other people, anorexics tended to adjust the picture until it quite accurately reflected that person's size, but when faced with a picture of themselves, they adjusted the picture so that it was significantly bigger than they actually were.[11]

There can be no doubt that severely ill anorexics do lose sight of how dreadfully skinny and emaciated they are, but some experts have questioned how genuinely subconscious this distortion of one's own body image is. One former sufferer from anorexia nervosa wrote to me saying that, 'Of course I knew how skinny I was, but I never said so. I knew that if I admitted anything they would think they had won. The psychiatrists would think there was a chink in my armour, and they would be able to get me to eat. But, believe me, I knew.'

123

There is simply no way of knowing how many anorexics are this aware of their problem. What does seem certain is that many anorexics have a terrible fear that they could overeat. Like alcoholics who have gone 'on the wagon' and worry that one drink will tilt them back into alcoholism, anorexics have a similar attitude to food: 'If I eat, will I be able to stop? Will I be able to control myself?'

What are the effects of anorexia?

The main physical effect of anorexia is the very obvious loss of weight. As a result of this, a number of other problems are almost inevitable and include over-sensitivity to cold, constipation, low blood pressure, a slow heart rate, and hypothermia. In addition to these, menstruation stops. I have briefly explained why periods stop, but another consequence of the low levels of oestrogen, the female sex hormone, in women with anorexia is that their bones may become less strong. Most people have now heard of the osteoporosis, or bone thinning, that can occur in women after the menopause. Not all anorexics are aware that they too can face the same problem, but at a much younger age. For this reason, hormone treatment can be of real value.

Curiously, it has been calculated that in approximately 10 to 20 per cent of people with anorexia nervosa, the periods stop *before* the weight loss has occurred. Periods usually re-start when the BMI (see Chapter 8) reaches 19, although in some they may start before this.

There is also an increased risk of infertility in women who have suffered from anorexia nervosa.

What is the Outlook in Anorexia Nervosa?

Obviously there isn't space in a book such as this to look at all the treatments available for anorexia nervosa, but suffice it to say that it is a condition that always requires professional help. With help, most sufferers do improve. The aims of treatment in anorexia are threefold:

- reaching a weight within a normal range (say, a BMI of over 19);
- eating normally, as compared to non-anorexics of comparable age and social class, without needing repeated and excessive diets; and
- developing sufficient self-knowledge, and a range of skills in coping with problems (including sexuality) so she no longer 'needs' the anorexia.

Using these criteria, probably seven out of ten anorexics will respond fully to treatment, though this may take a long time. Some of the others will continue to have eating problems, such as bulimia nervosa, and a small group will continue to have anorexia for many years. It is generally accepted that the older you are when anorexia nervosa develops, the worse the outlook tends to be. It is, however, never, ever hopeless.

But anorexia nervosa can kill. Experts estimate that the death rate is approximately 2 per cent, many of which may have taken an overdose of drugs.

Atypical Eating Disorders

There are quite a few women whose eating problems do not precisely fit the strict criteria for either bulimia or anorexia. How do you classify someone who behaves like an anorexic, but whose weight is above the level required for the diagnosis of anorexia nervosa? How do you label someone who binge eats only occasionally, rather than regularly?

The American Psychiatric Association, in the DSM-III manual, calls these problems 'Atypical Eating Disorders', and stresses that sufferers should be aware that they have a problem, that they have a preoccupation (like anorexics) with food, body size and dieting, and that the problem interferes with their everyday lives. Sometimes people with these problems are recovering from either bulimia or anorexia. Sometimes they may be on the first steps downwards. Either way, they do need specific help.

Atypical eating disorders can be remarkably common.

Among women aged between fifteen and thirty, and depending on the actual study performed, it is thought that something between 10 and 30 per cent may suffer from these problems. Nearly one-third of all young women may have at least one episode of disordered eating, and around about a quarter believe that their preoccupation with their body shape posed a problem for them.

Why Bother with These Sub-divisions Anyway?

As you have looked at these different types of eating disorders, it may have struck you that they actually have more features in common than they have differences. The real differences are between those with eating problems and those who eat 'normally'. So why do we bother with these sub-divisions and the problems that they pose?

It is certainly possible that in future, we may move away from trying to put people into diagnostic boxes, and instead will tailor specific therapies to the individual rather than groups, as already happens in much complementary medicine, and the best conventional medical care.[12] However, there is still some benefit in reasonably broad diagnostic categories. For instance, if you, or someone you care for, has been diagnosed as suffering from bulimia then this does give you an easy way of knowing where to look for help. Most of this book would not be of specific relevance to many sufferers from anorexia nervosa, but the label has, at least, given you the chance to know where and how to search for information. And information, knowledge and understanding are absolutely vital if you are going to begin to cope with eating disorders.

Men with Bulimia

Male bulimics have probably been feeling rather left out until now. The earlier chapters are as relevant to you, but since bulimia is so much more common in women, it seemed logical to concentrate on the female experience.

But bulimia does happen in males. Singer Elton John has reportedly been a sufferer in the past, and doubtless there are other celebrities who have not yet talked about it. After all, look at any open-shirted, bare-chested, rock 'n' roll singer and you will see that slim is in. I suspect it is only a matter of time before more male bulimics with a high-media profile come forward. And then it may be just a short step to more men in general owning up to their bulimia.

Of course, as we shall see in this chapter, there are plenty of reasons why more women suffer from bulimia, but this doesn't mean that women suffer more. For the individual male bulimic, the problems are every bit as bad. It is one thing to be isolated and alone when you suffer from a well-recognised condition. It is quite another to be isolated, alone, and to believe that you are something of a freak. And it also takes considerable courage to admit to something which has always been considered a woman's problem. The more the problem can be seen as one which affects both sexes, the more men will feel comfortable about seeking treatment.

How Common is Bulimia in Men?

The pressures to which I have just referred make it all the more difficult to know how common bulimia is in men. However, it has been estimated that bulimia affects approximately one man in four hundred between the ages of thirteen and thirty. In community studies, about one bulimic in ten will be male,[1] and the ratio of female to male sufferers has changed over the past five years from 50 to 1 to 30 to 1.

Bulimia nervosa tends to start at a later age in men than in women. Whereas the average age of onset for women is between fifteen and eighteen, in men the average age of onset is more likely to be between eighteen and twenty-six years. It is possible, though not certain, that this is simply a result of puberty generally happening later in boys than in girls.

Particular groups of men do seem to be more prone to bulimia nervosa. These include models, dancers, long-distance runners and men who are in occupations which emphasise body weight. There is also evidence that homosexuality is a contributing factor. Certainly a higher proportion of bulimic men than bulimic women are gay. It is also known that there is a higher than expected incidence of drug or alcohol abuse in male bulimics, in particular cocaine. Men who become bulimic are more likely to have been overweight previous to the illness than their female counterparts. However, in almost every other respect the male experience of bulimia is very similar to that of women.

Why are there fewer bulimic men than bulimic women?

How someone feels about their body can be tremendously important in determining whether they develop bulimia nervosa. In a study of British secondary school students it was found that the girls became progressively less and less satisfied with their body size and shape as they aged from eleven to eighteen, whereas the boys were, in general, unconcerned about their bodies.[3] Why should this be? In Chapter 7, we examined late twentieth-century Western society and its extraordinary obsession with slimness in women. But until recently, the pressures on men have been very different. Generally it has been far more acceptable for men to be overweight. Look at any TV series. Powerful men frequently have a paunch, while the female characters will be slim, unless they play a lesser role in the script. Male stars seem to come in all shapes and sizes. Think back to the male characters and actors who have exuded power and success despite being large – Brian Blessed, Robbie Coltrane or Peter Ustinov.

Indeed, the opposite has been true for many years. Think about the body-building courses that look down on the 'seven-stone weakling' who will have sand kicked in his face; the seaside postcard image of the little skinny man who is dominated by his wife; the television characters who use their thinness to portray an image of being a wimp, characters such as Sid Little of 'Little and Large', or even the tank-topped Frank Spencer as portrayed by Michael Crawford in 'Some Mothers Do Have 'Em'. Women who were this slim would be fashion models. But the men are wimps.

So, the image of excessively slim men has in the past been negative. The pressures on men to reach a state of extreme slimness didn't exist. However, there are other pressures, and these relate to fitness, to training and to body-building. In addition, the nature of society is changing. Ten years ago, naked male pin-ups in women's magazines were unheard of. Now they are becoming commonplace. Male pop groups regularly perform or pose shirtless for photographs. Colour supplements are full of advertisements featuring near-naked men, whether they are adverts for ice cream, aftershave or underarm deodorant. These men all have one thing in common – they might not be skinny, but they certainly don't have a hint of excess fat. Pure muscle and taut flesh is the order of the day. And for many men, the increased attention that is increasingly being paid to physique and fatness could easily be the trigger that takes them towards bulimia.

In July 1993, London's *Daily Express* ran a full-page story about some fascinating research conducted by psychologist Dr Jane Ussher, which showed that six out of ten men believe a change in body shape would make them healthier and more sexually attractive, and that three out of ten women dislike their partner's physique.[5] The study suggested that sexual identity for men was becoming more closely linked with body shape. As a result, it seems more than likely that men will get caught in the same eating disease traps as women. After all, over-strict dieting can be the first step into the dieting and bingeing cycle.

What may help to prevent this is the apparent biochemical differences between men and women mentioned in Chapter 8. It is known that an increased level of 5HT (see page 83) decreases the appetite. In a study of healthy women who were fed a restricted diet for four days followed by an episode of overfeeding, biochemical changes were noted which were directly linked to the amount of 5HT which could be produced in the central nervous system. While the women were on the controlled diet it was found that their potential for 5HT production was reduced, but in similar studies on men this did not happen. It seems as if the way in which dieting affects brain biochemistry is specific to women. As well as the pressing psychological and social pressures, it is also conceivable that this could explain why far fewer men suffer from bulimia.

There are other possible biological explanations as to why women develop bulimia more frequently than men. During the adolescent growth spurt, males tend to put on muscle whereas females put on fat. The development of the female curves, the result of fat being laid down, is embarrassing for many girls. In contrast, boys are usually happy to become bigger and more muscular. Normal adolescent development can be much more upsetting for girls than for boys.

It is also quite likely that men find dieting easier. This is simply because their metabolic rate tends to be somewhat higher, so a given level of calorie restriction will have a more profound effect. But psychology has an enormous effect when it comes to dieting, too. Many women want to be very thin, viewing thinness in a very positive light, but extreme thinness in males is seen negatively. The psychological brakes are likely to come on much sooner.

For this reason, male bulimics tend not to be quite as concerned about their binge eating as their female counterparts, and in general are not quite so desperate about strict control of their weight. But, as we shall see, real problems can still arise.

How does it feel to be a male with bulimia?

Barry wrote to me at length about his experiences. He had suffered from an eating disorder for nearly ten years, and as he said in his introduction:

> My main problem was one of body image linked with low self-esteem stemming from my parents, especially my mother who ceaselessly criticised me. I am also in regular contact with other males with eating problems. Each case is different, but all without fail have feelings of insecurity and confusion over their identity. Other males may turn to drink or drugs or domestic violence rather than anorexia or bulimia, and this must be why fewer males suffer from eating disorders. We just internalise our problems differently.

Barry began training at the age of fourteen. He felt good about his body, joined a weight-lifting club, and spent more and more of his time training. But things gradually turned sour:

> In the summer of 1976 my preoccupation with improving my body became obsessional. I had always dreamt of being big and muscular, but several people at college remarked that although I trained hard I didn't look good. I assumed that by this they meant that I was fat. So, I cut out the normal culprits – cakes, sweets and chocolates, and within a few weeks my body had shed fat! I felt great, and bought new clothes. This was obviously the way to go.

131

However, once the novelty wore off I tightened my diet even more. I started training for two hours a day, seven days a week. My diet consisted of high-protein, low-carbohydrate food (I shudder at the thought now), my body fat was around 6 per cent and I could actually see veins over my stomach.

During 1977 I realised I was becoming obsessional as a certain pattern of behaviour was emerging. I found that I could cope with life as long as I could train and eat as I had planned. If anything affected this ritual then I couldn't cope. My college work suffered as I just couldn't devote enough time to study.

I struggled through to summer of 1977 when I had to go on a fieldwork trip abroad. On this trip we had to walk up to fifteen miles a day. My body felt totally drained, and one morning I decided to eat a little more to try and combat my lack of energy. It worked, but at a price. I started to worry that I would get fat, so in addition to my walking activities I took up running. Thus I was in a ridiculous situation of eating more to help me, but then burning it up with extra activity.

One afternoon, after walking in the mountains I went into a cake shop and stuffed myself. I couldn't stop. I felt sick and disgusted with myself, but I just couldn't stop. I went to sleep feeling my body, testing for fat.

I awoke the next day in a state of sheer panic. I felt totally out of control. Somehow I managed to get home without eating any more 'bad food' but I then binged again. For the next few weeks I controlled my food during the week, and then binged at weekends. It was as though all the foods that I had deprived myself of during the previous year were shouting out at me.

This story will be familiar to so many bulimia sufferers, whether male or female, as will Barry's closing comments, 'I can honestly say that at this time I never felt happy. I trained to eat, and after I ate, I had to train. I didn't know where it was all going to end. I now realise that even if I had reached physical perfection, I would have never believed it as I was quite incapable of being happy and satisfied with myself.'

Barry did sort out his problems, and now spends a considerable amount of time talking to, and helping, other male bulimics. He is certain of one thing, 'If I had received some form of counselling to help me deal with my problems and insecurities, then I would never have suffered for so many years.'

If you are a male bulimic, then talk to someone. Follow the advice that I give in Part Four. Telephone the Eating Disorders Association, or talk to your doctor. But remember, *you are not alone*. There are many other male bulimics who know what you are going through. And one day you will even be able to do something that Barry thought he would never do. His letter finished quite simply 'P.S., I can now look in the mirror.'

BULIMIA CAN BE HELPED

Throughout this book I have highlighted the tremendous physical, psychological and sociological pressures that can cause and maintain bulimia. But the situation is not hopeless. Bulimia can be helped. If you suffer from bulimia, you have gone a long way towards sorting out your problems to be reading this far into the book. You are beginning to understand what is going on and why you feel the way that you do. If you care for someone with bulimia, this book should have helped you put the problem into context. It is probably nowhere near as straightforward as you first thought it. So many people see bulimia as simply a disease of vanity, a compulsion to be slim and attractive that gets out of hand. But, as you now realise, it is much more than that.

You may have read this far and have decided that you do not actually have full-blown bulimia nervosa, or that your problems are really not serious enough to seek further help or therapy. If this is the case, you may be right, but do be careful that you are not suffering from yet another effect of the low self-esteem that so affects people with bulimia. You may be feeling that your problems don't warrant attention, that compared to some of the case histories in this book they are trivial. But please remember that you do matter. However trivial you may believe your problems to be, if they bother you then they need to be solved. Talk to someone about them, to a self-help group, a friend, a doctor. But don't run away from sorting things out because you don't think you are significant enough.

Understanding bulimia is the first step on the path to recovery. This final section of the book will look at all the various aspects of treatment. I will examine the basic principles behind treatment, the forms of therapy that are available, the places of self-help, the role of organisations like the Eating Disorders Association, and the place of medication. If you are the relative or friend of someone with bulimia, I will show you how you can best help him or her recover. At the moment you may be feeling trapped by your bulimia, and worried that the situation is hopeless. Nothing could be further from the truth.

Finally, this section of the book is directed primarily at the person with bulimia. For this reason, the focus will be on what 'you' feel, rather than what 'someone with bulimia' feels. In Chapter 22 I will be highlighting more directly the concerns of carers.

15

Owning Up

You have already taken the first step in tackling your bulimia by finding out about the problem, about its complexities, causes and results. So far, so good, but things now have to become personal.

To begin with, ask yourself three simple questions:

- Do I want to get better?
- How much?
- Why?

These may seem too obvious. Doesn't everyone with bulimia want to get better? Well, everyone doesn't matter here. You do. Have you really decided that now is the time to begin to sort things out? Are you doing it because you are under pressure from family or friends, or is your heart really in it? The next weeks and months may not be easy, and it is vital that you have made a firm, personal and honest commitment.

Reading the earlier part of the book will have shown you that binge eating is not the problem. It is a symptom of the problems that you have with coping with stresses. Your stresses may be caused by emotional, family or relationship difficulties. They may be a result of boredom, of Pre-Menstrual Syndrome, of fear of the future, of your reluctance to take chances in case everything doesn't work out to be perfect. I know that you don't think very much of yourself at present, but I hope that you might gradually begin to like and respect yourself some more.

So, the next most important step is the apparently simple one of owning up. Admitting that you do have a problem, that your relationship with food and eating has become abnormal, and that you want to sort it out. I am well aware that there are all sorts of emotions tied up with making a decision like this. Despite the glamour that occasionally seems to be associated with bulimia – many high-profile and attractive people such as film stars have begun admitting to being bulimic – there is nevertheless still a tremendous stigma attached to the condition.

Even more of a problem may be involved in coming to terms with the feeling that I heard very clearly expressed by one woman with bulimia. 'I'd love to be helped,' she said. 'I mean, I really want to be treated, but I also want to stay slim and I'm terrified that dealing with the bulimia might make me less slim. Let's face it, I think at the moment I would rather be slim with bulimia, than be fat without it.' These fears are real, but the choice is not just between bulimia and slimness, as we will continue to see throughout this section.

You may feel ashamed of having bulimia. You may feel guilty. You already have little respect for yourself, and you may feel that owning up and admitting to anyone that you are bulimic may make them reject you. In fact, it is more likely that those who are close to you and who love you will have been aware for some time that things are not right, and will be thoroughly relieved to know what is going on. The unknown is always more frightening than a problem that is understood.

Do you remember Jane, the airline hostess whose story opened this book? Her bulimia became worse and worse.

> Every day would start out the same, trying to be better, trying to be good, but this thing had got the better of me.

Her story continues:

> One night I was watching TV with the family and we

were having a family debate which got a bit heated. I just absolutely broke down crying and ran upstairs. My mum came up and asked what was wrong, and it all came out about the ugly double life I was leading. Once I had admitted my problem to my mum it was like acknowledging the problem to myself for the first time in my life. The tears flowed all night long, and I knew I needed help.

Of course, some people do become aware of their own bulimia at a very early stage, and are able to deal with it rapidly and relatively simply. Their eating disorder may still just be an occasional problem, and may not have become a habit. However, for the majority, the onset is insidious. You may have started out simply having the occasional binge. So what? So do many people. There's nothing too unusual about that. But at some stage over the past few months or years you will have realised that the problem has really become out of control.

You will have gradually begun to use food as a means of dealing with your stress. When you feel like bursting, when you feel that life is simply too much, then you binge. An essential reason for admitting your bulimia to someone else is that your main way of dealing with stress is also the problem. Are you really going to be able to sort out the stress of bulimia by yourself, without using it as a prop to help you through? You need to realise that your biggest prop will have gone. I will be teaching you other ways of coping with stress, but do not underestimate the pressures that you may be under. It really will be worth it.

And since you have come this far, do decide to sort out your problems now. Don't wait. Your bulimia is most unlikely to go away by itself. The longer that the vicious cycle is kept in motion, the more you will be trapped inside it, and the more reluctant you will be to escape.

It's important that you should talk to someone, and in the next chapter I will look at some of the different professionals and groups who might help you. Sharing your problem with someone will come as a great relief.

While a problem shared becomes much less frightening,

it still remains a problem until you have uncovered its roots and prevented any further growth. As a doctor, I know how many people believe that by talking to me their problems become my responsibility. This happens repeatedly in the area of obesity. I well remember a lady with severe obesity telling a local shopkeeper about how useless she thought I was at helping her lose weight. He thought it was really quite funny, as his shop is the local fish and chip shop and she'd been complaining over a large portion of pie and chips. Once she had consulted me, she had seen the problem as being partially mine, and her responsibility to have been reduced.

Whoever you tell, however many people become involved in helping you, your bulimia remains your problem. At the end of the day, it is you who are going to sort it out. Help will be there, but it is you who must take responsibility for yourself. Involving others is not a way of passing the problem to them. It is more a way of signalling to yourself and to others that you are taking this problem seriously, and may need some help along the way.

And, important though it has been to discuss the causes of bulimia, it is a total waste of your time to blame others for what has happened. You may be a victim of your family, or of society, but you can only live forwards. The past has finished. You do have control over what happens now. Thousands of bulimics have trodden this path before you.

Why Is It Worth Getting Better?

After highlighting some of the problems that you may be going to face, it is also pertinent to ask why you should bother. Aren't you getting by as you are? Is the possible pain really going to be worth it? In reality, very few sufferers are happy about being bulimic. Pleasure with bulimia rarely lasts long. It is true that at an early stage many people echo Lynn Redgrave's words on discovering self-induced vomiting as a means of counter-acting her need for binges. 'I discovered an amazingly easy way out,' she wrote. 'I started throwing up . . . It seemed like the perfect solution.'[1] But this pleasant surprise is replaced by disgust, guilt and despair.

Let's consider the following benefits of beating bulimia.

Health reasons
In Chapter 5 I dealt in some detail with the various health hazards that are associated with bulimia. In summary, the following parts of the body and its systems can be affected:

- teeth and gums – tooth decay and ulceration;
- salivary glands – swelling;
- throat – persistent soreness and damage;
- oesophagus – acid reflux, long-term damage at the stomach junction;
- abdomen – pain and swelling;
- anus – irritation and soreness;
- skin – dry skin and hair;
- electrolyte disturbances;
- heart and circulation – irregular beats and palpitations;
- menstrual disturbances;
- swollen feet and ankles; and
- kidney damage and urinary infections.

It's quite a frightening list; however, with the notable exception of the damage caused to teeth from stomach acid, almost all of these are reversible.

Finally, while considering the physical reasons for dealing with your bulimia, it is important not to forget childbearing. At some stage you may wish to have children. Unlike anorexia, bulimia does not appear to interfere with fertility, and so it is all the more important to have the problem behind you when eventually you choose to have children. In particular, you need to be avoiding purging and vomiting at this time as it interferes with healthy nutrition, and can cause electrolyte imbalances. If, indeed, you are pregnant please be honest and talk about your bulimia to your doctor or midwife right away.

Social reasons
Bulimia is probably playing havoc with your social life. Much social interaction revolves around eating and drinking: socialising at work takes place at coffee breaks; going out for a meal is a popular way of getting to meet people. The problems that you have with food not only make this sort of occasion something to dread, and certainly find hard to enjoy, but the sheer practicalities of, for instance, having to excuse yourself to find a toilet somewhere to be able to vomit, can cause you real distress.

And bulimia worsens your feelings of poor self-esteem. You don't like yourself very much, and are bound to think that others will feel the same. Feelings like guilt, self-disgust and shame do not lead to successful or happy social situations. Sorting out your bulimia will help your self-respect more than you'd ever believe.

Psychological reasons
Wouldn't it be good to like yourself again? To be able to mix happily with people? To be able to wake in the morning thinking about the everyday worries and pleasures faced by the majority of the human race, rather than being totally obsessed with food, diet and the shape of your body?

You may be wondering if you can ever regain these good feelings. After all, you may be thinking, if your bulimia has resulted from your poor self-esteem and other psychological problems, then how can sorting out your bulimia ever do more than just put you back to square one? Well, it can. Simply facing up to and beating the bulimia will give you a tremendous sense of pride and satisfaction. These may be feelings that you have never experienced before. Take my word for it, they will do you good!

Why am I saying it is going to be so difficult?

I am aware that you may find some of what I have written in this chapter worrying. However, I do believe that it is important to realise the scale of the task that you are taking on. That doesn't mean that it's not going to be worth it. In fact, the opposite applies. The fact that it's not likely to be easy makes it even more worthwhile.

To begin with, you will be throwing away your psychological crutch at the very time that you feel most in need of it. Secondly, there is the problem that, without help, you are likely to resist bingeing by putting yourself on a diet, and we have already seen that dieting is the very thing that is most likely to drive you to bingeing again. Dieting is part of the problem: most dieters spend a huge amount of time thinking about food, just about the last thing that you need to be doing. Most people who try and sort out their own bulimia do the very thing that is most likely to trigger the problem.

There is also a big difference between coming to terms with a problem like bulimia and one like giving up smoking or drinking. You can survive without nicotine or alcohol. You cannot survive without food. Several times every day you are going to have to deal with the very thing that gives you problems. You may be concerned that by retraining your eating habits, and abandoning the purging, vomiting and dieting, then you'll end up being extremely overweight. It will not happen: getting into a normal eating pattern gets rid of the pressures to binge. Bulimics eat enormous amounts, then diet. Normal eating stops the former and negates the need for the latter.

As a result of some of these stresses, many people who begin to tackle their bulimia feel severely depressed. This is usually worse at the start, and eases as time goes on. But be aware that it may happen. You may experience many other unusual feelings, too – like anxiety, fear and loneliness – which you have been keeping suppressed. All your emotions have been muffled by the bulimia – don't be frightened when they begin to make themselves heard. They are a sign that you are coming to life again. Soon you will be feeling good again. Instead of getting by from day to day, with your very existence determined by your relationship to food, you will be back in the world of everyday joys and sadness, laughter and tears. Emotions are not a bad thing.

It is all going to be worth it. The next chapter will tell you who can help you, and I will go on to discuss such areas as medication, the ways in which you can help yourself, and how to look after yourself once the bulimia has come under control. I will also highlight alternative ways of learning to cope with stress which will save you from having to use bulimia to help you get through.

As one woman who had lived with bulimia for years wrote to me:

> Please do encourage your readers to sort themselves out. For me, tackling the eating problem was the best thing that I have ever done. I now look back on my days with bulimia with real sadness. It all seems such a waste. But now that I have come through and understand myself so much better, I feel a new woman. Please tell them. It really is worth it.

16

The Aims of Treatment

Most people with bulimia will have tried to sort themselves out. They will have resolved to stop bingeing. They will have almost inevitably put themselves on a diet. Sadly, as a result of both the psychological and physiological pressures that the dieting causes, the pressure to binge again will have continued to build up until it bursts in an orgy of bingeing. Back you go to square one, demoralised and apparently defeated.

So, before tackling your bulimia you need to have a clear idea of what the aims of treatment are. These are best summarised as follows:

- learning to change your eating behaviour;
- dealing with your excessive concern about body size and weight; and
- learning to cope with your feelings – without resorting to bulimia.

In the next few chapters I will be looking at the various ways in which you might go about tackling these; at the end of the day it's up to you to reach these aims, whether by yourself or with professional help. While some people with bulimia are able to deal with the problem almost entirely by themselves, or with the very minimum of support, it is fair to say that not everyone is able, or should even necessarily try, to sort out their own problems.

I am particularly concerned about people who feel that

they are totally alone in their struggle. If you are emotionally isolated you will find self-help too much of a struggle. Even if you only begin by talking to an Eating Disorders Association (see page 216) contact over the phone, I am certain that you do need someone to share your feelings and experiences with.

Secondly, people suffering from anorexia nervosa and who have a very low body weight in addition to their bulimia nervosa, also need professional help, as do those with other significant psychological or physical problems. If you are suicidal at times then I would urge you to talk to a professional.

Let's look at the various aims of treatment in a little more detail.

Learning to change your eating behaviour

The ultimate aim here is for you eventually to treat food and eating in the same way as the majority of 'normal' eaters. This is probably the best, or at least the simplest, definition of normality. Most people are not terribly controlled and obsessional about their eating. They eat an average of three meals a day, which is something to aim for.

Most people don't count calories all the time. They eat what they fancy without feeling guilty about it. Sometimes they eat too much, and sometimes they skip meals. Without food ruling their every waking moment, their lives go on.

Rule number one is that normal eating does not involve diet books. It also means abandoning the concept of 'good' and 'bad' foods. There are no such things. The entire multi-national massive slimming and dieting industry does nothing but promote this concept, but they are wrong, and we have already seen how much harm they do.

Try this experiment. Write down a list of the foods that you think of as being 'bad'. When you have done that, move on.

Now look at the list that you have produced. Does it look familiar? It probably looks very much like a list of the foods that you binge on. By terming these foods as 'bad' they somehow become more tempting. It is also completely impossible to avoid all of them all the time. If you eat one of them, a biscuit for example, you may feel that you have been weak, and that you've lost control of your diet.

It is absolutely essential that eventually you start to eat all types of food in moderation. Even those demons on your personal list.

Don't worry if this all seems extraordinary, and simply too much to take in. I will suggest some ways of coping.

Food is meant to be enjoyable: sustenance, nourishment, comfort and pleasure. It should not, however, control you, and it is not something about which you need to be obsessed. I hope that you will even be able to go out for a meal in a restaurant and eat and enjoy the same food, in the same quantities, that everyone with you is eating.

Finally, remember that 'dieting' simply doesn't work. I have discussed many reasons why this should be, but just ignore all the science for a minute and think about the topic logically. If 'dieting' – by which I mean calorie controlled dieting – really worked then the slimming industry would be getting smaller rather than bigger. If books on losing weight worked, then there wouldn't be any need for any more books on the topic.

Indeed, agents for one of the Very Low Calorie diets, which involve people substituting sachets of soups or milk-shake for meals, find that if they contact former clients about 9 to 15 months after their last purchase, they can almost always sell them fresh supplies as the weight will have gone back on again.

If food meant only nutrition to human beings then it would be simple to cut down and lose weight. But it doesn't. Food means much more, and without recognising this fact, calorie-counting will always fail. That's why dieting is a disaster. Don't even try it. (For advice on healthy eating see chapter 20.)

Dealing with your excessive concern about body size and weight

Every day the same thoughts go through your mind and you worry about your weight. Many bulimics weigh themselves several times a day. They glance at themselves in mirrors, shop windows, car windows, and almost anything shiny to see if they can gauge how overweight they look. Some bulimics do exactly the opposite. They are so certain that their appearance will revolt them that they do everything in their power to avoid their reflection.

Neither one of these behaviours is healthy, and that is all part of your problem. When you put your bulimia behind you, you'll have no need for this. At present you probably believe that if you don't keep a check on your weight and size then everything will rapidly drift out of control. This simply is not true.

It is time to determine what your correct weight should be. Healthy weight is usually determined by looking at your height. If I ask you to say what weight you would like to be, you are likely to name a weight that is substantially below the ideal weight as shown on standard height and weight charts. In fact, a large proportion of women, whether bulimic or not, are wholly dissatisfied with their actual weight and would like to be anything up to a stone and a half lighter. But if you set your target weight too low, then the only way in which you will be able to reach it will be by excessive dieting, which will just initiate the starve-binge cycle problems again. It's important to be realistic.

In Chapter 7 I explained the concept of the BMI (Body Mass Index). This shows you the range of ideal weights for your height, and it would certainly be useful to see where your current target weight features. However another definition of a normal weight is simply the weight at which your body would settle if you are eating and exercising normally. Most of the human race do not end up obese. They level out at a weight which stays pretty steady and

148

is determined by a combination of their metabolism, and their energy intake and expenditure.

Having a low target weight has all sorts of spin-offs. You are likely to buy clothes that are actually too tight for your normal weight. The discomfort is a constant reminder that you are dissatisfied with yourself. Why not buy comfortable clothes?

People with bulimia vary dramatically in how they deal with their weight. Maybe you weigh yourself several times a day – on to the scales as soon as you wake – in the knowledge that your weight is usually lowest in the morning. On to the scales at any other opportunity during the day – after a meal, after going to the toilet, after exercising, after bingeing or purging – any time at all, simply to see what changes there have been. Alternatively you may steer clear of scales at all times. Who knows what terrible message they might have for you?

The simple fact is that everyone's weight varies considerably from hour to hour, from day to day. Frequently these changes mean nothing. Often they have little to do with the amount of fat in your body, and far more to do with the amount of fluid. But there is a danger that if the scales say that you have lost a pound or two, you may feel unjustified pleasure and pride which is bound to be deflated when your weight shifts back up again. If you find you have gained weight, this is exactly the sort of depressing upset that may drive you into binge eating. It is almost as if you have been using your weight and your size and shape as a measure of your own value. Perhaps in future you will be able to value yourself simply for being the person that you are.

But to ignore your weight totally would probably cause you too much strain, and as I am advising and encouraging you to eat in a new and different way then I think it is important that you keep an eye on progress.

Weigh yourself naked, first thing in the morning, on one day each week. Do not weigh yourself at any other time. Daily fluctuations really don't mean anything at all, but a weekly weigh-in will give you an accurate guide to how your revised eating and exercising habits are affecting you. Make sure your scales are accurate and consistent. If you get on, off, and back on a set of scales it should read the same on each occasion.

If you are in the habit of weighing yourself umpteen times a day, then you may need to wean yourself from this addiction. Cut down slowly, first to maybe two or three times a day, then daily, then on alternate days, then twice a week, and eventually weekly. Sticking to a weekly weigh-in is essential. If you decide to have an extra weigh-in mid-week, there is a real risk that this meaningless extra reading could so upset you that it could trigger the bingeing.

Finally, many people use exercise to help control their size and shape. If your sole reason for exercising is keeping slim, then abandon it. Find something that you can enjoy. Exercise that is just there to do you good is something that will either become an unhealthy obsession, or is something that you will abandon. Do something you enjoy. There are plenty of alternatives out there: cycling, swimming, badminton, tennis, gardening, dancing, step classes and walking the dog. You don't have to own a tracksuit and pair of expensive trainers to get exercise. But make it fun.

Learning to cope with your feelings – without resorting to bulimia

We have already seen how very closely binge eating and other bulimic activity is linked to the way that you feel. Not only are people who come from families who find it difficult to express their emotions more likely to be bulimic, but bulimics also tend to have the low self-esteem that is more likely to create in them a feeling of stress.

Dealing with stress is of fundamental importance in tackling your bulimia. This will form an important part of the rest of the book, and I will cover the various ways in which you might get help. But, please remember, I am not showing you how to suppress your emotions. Nor am I pretending that you will live in a stress-free world. What I want you to do is to acknowledge your feelings, and to find a way of expressing them without resorting to your old ally, bulimia. There are much better ways of getting through life.

17

The Types of Treatment

There is no single guaranteed cure for bulimia. How could there be? With a problem that is as complex as bulimia nervosa, with such a mixture of causes, triggers and spinners, it would be quite extraordinary if a single approach worked for everyone. In addition, different patients have different preferences for treatment. Some make it clear that they would never consider taking medication. Others find group therapy totally unacceptable. Still others never get the hang of some forms of psychotherapy. Treatment has to be matched to the individual.

As a result, there are numerous ways in which you can tackle your bulimia. These vary from simple self-help techniques, through medical or psychological treatment, the use of medication, psychotherapy and group therapy. This chapter will look briefly at some of the various alternatives that are available, and the various groups of people who can offer you help.

> Once I had told my mother about my bulimia I
> felt a great weight off my mind. I suppose I hadn't
> really owned up to myself before then. But at last I
> realised I needed help. I wanted to be helped. Before
> then, no one had been able to get through to me. I
> had read articles and things about bulimia, of course,
> but none of it had really made an impact. Yes, I had
> taken it on board on one level, but it was only when
> I really accepted that I, me, myself, was the one with

bulimia, not someone I was reading about, that I was ready to be helped. I suddenly felt that I needed a lot of help. And I wanted it straight away. What had been a problem for some years suddenly became an emergency. Melanie, bank clerk, aged 24.

Of course, not everyone with bulimia needs specialist help. If your problem is relatively minor, you may be able to sort it out fairly quickly and easily by yourself – as long as you continue to take note of the advice and suggestions in this book. In Chapter 19 I will be looking at a method of self-help that many people with bulimia find tremendously beneficial. This may be all that you need. However, I do believe that almost everyone needs support. If you are going to tackle the problem by yourself, confide in someone. It could be someone in your family, a good friend, a telephone contact from the Eating Disorders Association (see page 216), or your doctor. Your own doctor should be happy to talk to you and to see you regularly for support while you tackle the self-help measures I outline here.

This chapter looks at the various sources of help that are available to you.

Doctors

Most doctors are part of an increasingly large primary healthcare team, consisting of nurses, health visitors, physiotherapists, administrative staff and so on. You may have known your doctor for many years, or alternatively he or she may be a complete stranger. Inevitably doctors vary tremendously in their knowledge of eating disorders, but even if they know next to nothing, they are still the gatekeepers to the other services available in the health industry.

In a typical week a family doctor will be dealing with problems ranging from sore throats to cancer, from unhappiness to schizophrenia, and from heart disease to diabetes, asthma or deafness. No doctor can possibly be an expert in everything, but even if he or she cannot help you directly, your family doctor should be able to put you in touch with someone who can. Doctors certainly should be experts in people, in understanding how your problem affects you as an individual, and one of the trademarks of a good family doctor is that he or she should be able to listen and make it safe and easy for you to talk and unburden your problems.

Doctors receive a large number of magazines and journals every week, and an increasing number of articles on eating disorders have been published in recent months. For instance, in the UK, one glossy weekly, *General Practitioner*, recently carried a five-page supplement devoted specifically to anorexia and bulimia, and in the same week three other magazines and medical journals carried specific articles on eating disorders and how to help them. Interest in these conditions is certainly growing.

As a family doctor for many years, I can suggest a few ways to make that first consultation about your bulimia as fruitful as possible. Ask the reception staff if you can have a double-length appointment. You should say that you have a complicated matter that you want to discuss, but under no circumstances should you have to tell the receptionist any more than that. Some practices will be happy to offer the extra time. Others will be reluctant. Either way, it is still worth asking.

Secondly, jot down a few notes about what you want to say and ask. You are bound to be nervous, and there is nothing more infuriating than getting home and only then remembering what you wanted to say.

Don't necessarily expect everything to be sorted out at once. With complex problems such as bulimia some doctors will just listen, and then suggest a further appointment. This is entirely reasonable. Many bulimics find the first consultation terribly stressful, and they may well not be in a receptive frame of mind for further discussion.

Unfortunately, a few doctors may appear totally uninterested in your problem. I would like to think that this is only a minority, but some may tell you to pull yourself together, or that bulimia is not a problem that they can help you with. They may even offer you a prescription almost before you've finished talking. If this

154

happens, consult a different doctor. You may find a more helpful doctor within the same practice, or you may have to change practices altogether. However, do give the doctor a chance. People with bulimia tend to have pretty dreadful self-esteem, and not only do they not like themselves very much, but they are at risk of assuming everyone else feels the same way. Don't go in on the defensive. Whatever you do, don't withdraw into your shell. You've taken a big step in seeking help. Don't stop now.

Changing doctors

In the UK you can choose to be registered with any doctor, and you do not have to give any reason why you are changing doctors. The new doctor is not necessarily obliged to take you on – for instance, his or her list may be full – but there should be no problem.

The best way to choose a new doctor is by personal recommendation. Ask family, friends or colleagues whom they recommend. In particular you want someone who has the ability to listen to problems. When choosing a doctor it is worth checking out their qualifications, which should be available from all practices. You should also find a local directory of doctors in your library. In Britain, doctors who have the qualifications MRCGP or FRCGP have taken the specialist examination of the Royal College of General Practitioners, and the Consumers' Association would recommend that you look out for a doctor with one of these qualifications.

If you cannot find a doctor to take you on, contact your local authority or health board. You will also find a list of local doctors in the Yellow Pages. But whatever you do, keep trying until you find someone who will help. A good doctor really is invaluable when it comes to sorting out your problems.

In a survey of members of the Eating Disorders Association (see page 216), only 43 per cent found their doctors to be particularly helpful in dealing with anorexia nervosa and bulimia. While this might seem disappointingly low, it was a level of satisfaction that applied to most other types of help as well.[1] Hopefully, as interest and knowledge about the condition grows, satisfaction levels will rise.

Janet told me about her doctor:

> I could see that she was a bit lost. She didn't seem to know much about bulimia, though it was a few years ago now, so I don't suppose many people did. However it was obvious that she really cared and wanted to help. She saw me regularly, and never once criticised me. She even phoned around various specialists to find the best one to help me further. I really did appreciate everything she did, though I suspect she thought she was pretty useless. Just knowing that she was there, and that I could see her and talk to her made all the difference.

Specialist Help

You may find that your family doctor has both the experience and the expertise to treat and advise you him or herself, particularly if your condition is relatively mild. However, it is quite likely that you will be referred on to a hospital or community-based specialist. If services are available, and your doctor suggests a referral, then do take advantage of the help that is on offer. One community therapist told me, 'One reason that things sometimes go wrong, and people even sometimes end up needing to be admitted to hospital, is that they have left everything too late. Entrenched patterns of behaviour are much harder to work with, and early referral to psychologists and trained nurses for a structured approach is considered essential by many of us.' If you are ready, willing and able to accept help – please do at the earliest possible opportunity.

If you live in an area where there is a specialist eating disorders clinic, then you may be referred directly there. Alternatively, your doctor may refer you to a member of your local mental health team. Again, depending on the area, your exact problem, and the expertise of the different team members, you may initially see a psychiatrist, a psychologist or a psychiatric nurse.

Not everyone needs highly specialised care, which is probably just as well. After all, a major survey published in 1993 showed that in the UK there were then just twenty-one specialist centres for eating disorders. These were units where at least twenty-five new patients with eating disorders were treated each year.[2] There are large areas of the country where there is no specialist centre, and others where patients had been refused access to the specialist centres that exist.

However, a report by a group of specialists stated that mild to moderate eating problems can be dealt with by family doctors, with the support of therapists and self-help groups. More severe problems (which includes the majority of cases of bulimia) should have more specialised care from a team lead by a local consultant psychiatrist with an interest in this type of problem, backed up by a full team of therapeutic and support services.

This form of 'stepped care' is ideal for eating disorders. Depending on the severity of problem, different levels of help and care should be available.[3] The more severe your problem, the more specialised the care that you require. Like many other medical problems, if any condition is mild, you help yourself. If it is more severe, you seek medical help. If your doctor can sort out the problem, he or she will. If not, you will see a local specialist, and if the problem is unusually severe you will need to see a regional or national specialist.

As bulimia varies so much from person to person, a variety of specific treatment levels have been suggested.[3] These are:

Level 1.   self-help, and self-help groups;
Level 2.   simple dietary advice on eating regularly, not eating alone, and not avoiding 'forbidden foods';
Level 3.   group counselling and therapy – perhaps once a week;
Level 4.   cognitive behaviour therapy (see page 159);

157

Level 5.   intensive group therapy (probably as a day patient); and
Level 6.   in-patient treatment – only needed rarely.

Wanting to be helped

There is one fundamental rule in all these therapies which is worth reiterating. If they are going to succeed, then you really must want to get better. Any therapist who helps you works from a position of equality, working *with* you against the problem. The therapist does not take the place of a concerned or caring parent, or loved one. The therapist becomes a tool that empowers you, that gives you help towards positive change. No therapist is there to twist your arm, to tell you what to do. You have to want to be helped before a helper can begin to help you. If you aren't ready for this, then you do have some more important thinking to do.

Different Forms of Therapy

In Chapter 18 I will be looking at the use of medication in treating bulimia. However the vast majority of therapies used in bulimia are 'talking therapies'. Even if you do have medication, some level of psychotherapy is still essential. You only have to look back at some of the triggering factors for bulimia to realise that increased self-awareness, increased self-confidence, and learning ways to cope with stress without using bulimia are essential to your recovery. If medication does help you, if you haven't dealt with these other problem areas in your life then when you stop the medication there is a real risk that you could drift back to your old habits and feelings.

By psychotherapy I do not mean psychoanalysis.

The forms of psychotherapy that are of value to people with bulimia are:

- cognitive therapy;
- supportive psychotherapy;
- behaviour therapy; and also

- relaxation therapy.

Cognitive therapy

Over the past few years, cognitive therapy has become one of the most promising and exciting developments in psychotherapy. Certainly the results in treating bulimia nervosa are extremely promising, with around 90 per cent of binge eaters reporting success in controlling this symptom.

It involves teaching people to think differently about their problems, so that their behaviour changes too. It really has two main functions in bulimia. One is to help people come to terms with their over-concern with their weight and size, and to learn to take a more realistic view of their appearance. In addition, it can help people deal with some of the stresses, such as depression and anxiety, that can trigger episodes of bingeing and purging. We have already seen that many people with bulimia feel that they are victims. Their self-confidence is low. Anything that happens to them is viewed negatively.

In cognitive therapy you will learn how to spot when you are automatically shifting into negative ways of thinking, and will be shown how you can re-interpret your feelings and problems more positively. You will learn how very many of your thoughts and fears are actually irrational, and can be countered by an alternative, more positive viewpoint. Instead of 'I need to be perfect and admired by everyone', you could think, 'No one is perfect. No one pleases everybody all the time. I need to be more realistic.' If you become more realistic, you are far less likely to be disappointed.

A typical exercise in cognitive therapy would be that whenever you feel yourself thinking negatively, you should write down the reason why. You can then look at the possible explanations for the situation. Realise that many of your fears have no basis in fact. Frequently people panic when they think of the consequences of what they have done, and become distressed and depressed about this. In fact, your fears may have so many 'ifs' that they are totally unrealistic.

Janice was worried about her young son, two-year-old Mark. She found Mark was an impossible handful. He would rarely behave as she wanted, and she felt she was losing control. She was terrified that other people would find out, that the social services would be informed, that they would judge her incompetent, that Mark would be put in care, that her husband would leave her, and so on, and on. A more realistic interpretation of events was that almost all mothers find two-year-olds dreadfully hard work and that she was coping every bit as well as anyone else.

But then Janice didn't think much of herself. She assumed everyone else was coping better, and the trail of 'ifs' in her fantasies about the results of her failure left her certain she would be childless and divorced. Recognising the way that her negative thinking dragged her down and learning ways of countering it helped Janice enormously. It also saved her from continuing to binge and purge as the release from her stress. Basic self-help cognitive therapy will be examined in Chapter 19.

Cognitive therapy is highly effective in the treatment of bulimia nervosa.[4] Typically, it takes between four and six months, and the therapist sees his or her clients on an individual basis. It is thought that, in the short term at least, about nine out of ten people will be helped to reduce their bingeing, and it seems likely that the improvement is permanent.

However, while cognitive behavioural therapy is the ideal treatment for bulimia nervosa, there are a minority of patients who do not respond to this at all. One study showed that this group was likely to have a longer history of bulimia, a greater level of laxative abuse than average, to have more severe depressed moods, and greater dissatisfaction with their body weight. They were also more likely to have abused psychoactive drugs, attempted to harm themselves, and have a lower self-esteem. There seems little doubt that people with bulimia in this group need

160

a much more intensive level of treatment than standard out-patient cognitive therapy can offer.[5]

Supportive Psychotherapy

Supportive psychotherapy – which may be used by doctors as well as local mental health experts – is used to help people through the crisis of coming to terms with their bulimia. Patients are encouraged to talk about their problems while the therapist listens sympathetically, and sometimes offers specific advice and even practical help.

This is more than what you would expect to achieve by talking things over with a friend. A skilled therapist will enable you to unload your feelings of guilt, fear and worry to a far greater extent. You will have undivided attention and concern for the duration of the therapy session.

Supportive psychotherapy also uses the technique of prestige suggestion. While normally the patient is specifically encouraged to take responsibility for her actions, and to work out solutions to her problems, the therapist may also confirm to the patient that she will be okay, that she will recover. This suggestion is not used often; after all, it is essential that the patient develops confidence herself and this makes it essential that she sorts out most of her problems herself. However, when confidence is crumbling, a firm reassurance from a skilled therapist can help bolster sagging spirits and allow improvement to continue.

Behaviour therapy

Whilst cognitive therapy is probably the mainstay of psychological treatment in bulimia, most therapists use a combination of cognitive and behavioural techniques. Traditional behaviour therapy itself relies on two main ideas – that exposure to something that you fear under safe conditions will make it less threatening, and that desirable behaviour can be encouraged using a system of rewards.

Looked at from a contemporary perspective, some of

the initial ideas of behaviour therapy developed earlier in the century might seem cruel and even brutal. Quite simply, good behaviour was rewarded and bad behaviour was discouraged. However, in the late 1960s and early 1970s, behaviour therapy began to evolve into cognitive behaviour therapy, where the impact of the way in which we think was considered in far more detail.

Behaviour therapy can be broken down into simple and complex techniques. Considering the more simple concepts first, behavioural study would highlight the basic way a person functions. In this way, social mixing ability, social skills (including assertiveness), levels of activity, eating habits, sleeping habits, ability to solve problems and obsessional behaviour are compared with appropriate 'normal' behaviour in those categories.

Some more complex behavioural techniques may also be used in bulimia. In such therapies, the therapist may encourage sufferers to accept that they may feel a strong urge to binge, but will also encourage them to prevent themselves from vomiting. Not being able to vomit makes the sufferer intensely anxious, and they then learn to cope with and deal with this anxiety. In this way the binge/purge cycle can be broken.

Rewarding good behaviour is another potentially valuable behavioural technique. This involves the person with bulimia rewarding herself appropriately for success. Bulimic sufferers frequently believe that their difficulties in controlling their problem are a sign of weakness, a defect in their character. They view themselves as weak willed, and they expect failure when they try to sort out the problem. Bulimia sufferers are therefore encouraged in therapeutic sessions, and also through diary keeping, to re-evaluate their successes and make adjustments to their own expectations. In this way they are slowly encouraged to restore or build a system of self-belief. Gradually their self-esteem improves, and as a result, their mood tends to pick up, and the cycle of bulimia can be dealt with.

In examining emotions, cognitive behaviour therapists frequently use a concept known as the three-system model of emotion. It sounds complicated, but is very logical and sensible. This says that in any given situation we are affected by:

system 1.   the way we think in that situation;
system 2.   the way we feel in that situation; and
system 3.   the way we behave in that situation.

Any one of these has influence on the other two. In other words, the way we feel affects the way we behave, and our beliefs. The way we behave affects our beliefs and feelings. And so on.

Psychological therapy can work on any of these different areas. The therapist can help deal with your approach to the problem, looking at the way society has affected your beliefs – rational and irrational – and your self-esteem. Or feelings may be targeted, teaching you how to cope with the negative feelings that bulimia may cause in you – feelings of panic, distress, breathlessness, and so on. Finally your actual behaviour can be the target.

One example of the way behaviour may be dealt with in the treatment of bulimia may involve some of the obsessional behaviours that you might have developed. Perhaps you constantly need and seek reassurance about your body shape, your weight, your looks. Perhaps you constantly check on these – looking in mirrors, jumping on the scales numerous times each day. Perhaps you are constantly asking yourself what people think of you. A cognitive behavioural therapist will tackle these, helping you to face them, and the emotions and thoughts that these behaviours cause.

The three different areas of emotion are obviously not truly separate. Help in any one area inevitably helps to unwind the problem in the others. In the same way as a vicious cycle can spiral downwards, do does improvement help you spiral back up.

Relaxation Therapy

Relaxation therapy may be combined with any of the

other forms of psychotherapy. The three-system model of emotions that I discussed on page 163 will have shown you how your feelings of stress will affect both your thoughts about yourself, and also your behaviour. It is obviously vital to learn how to deal with stress. None of us can ever live in a world without stress – we would probably die of boredom if we did – so rather than avoiding it, we should learn ways of coping. There are many simple techniques that can be learnt, and I will cover these in more detail in Chapter 20. At the moment you probably deal with stress by bingeing. Obviously, you will have far less need for this when you are able to use alternatives.

Hospital admission

Very few people with bulimia need to be admitted to hospital. After all, an essential part of dealing with bulimia involves learning to cope with the real world. If you are in hospital there is a real risk that you will come to rely on the staff and over-dependency on others becomes a very real problem.

Occasionally, of course, hospital admission is essential. It may be that the physical damage caused by bulimia has become very severe, or that there is some other associated illness, either physical or psychiatric. It may be that the individual is severely and suicidally depressed. A short stay may occasionally enable therapists to get to know the individual bulimia sufferer better, or to break a vicious cycle of problems that is being aggravated by the home environment. People with severe bulimia that has not been helped by prolonged out-patient therapy may also need admission, as may sufferers who live in very remote areas. Nevertheless, for the vast majority of people with bulimia, out-patient care is by far the most appropriate.

This chapter has only looked briefly at some of the techniques that may be used to help you deal with your bulimia. Every bulimic will receive treatment that is individual to her personal set of symptoms, triggers and spinners. I have only attempted to give you a flavour of what may happen. The good news is that most people with bulimia can be helped.

Drug Treatment

If part of the cause of bulimia is biochemical, then the question of whether it can be treated with medication is an important one. In Chapter 8 I discussed some of the current theories about the way that two particular chemicals, *serotonin* and *tryptophan*, may affect the bulimic.

As an understanding of how serotonin works is of great importance to this chapter, let me briefly summarise the biochemical theory involving these two key amino acids.

Tryptophan is an essential amino acid, and is important in hunger control. Many people on strict diets report that they feel depressed, and it has been shown that they also tend to have lower levels of tryptophan in their bloodstream. After eating food, particularly carbohydrates, the pancreas releases insulin, which increases the blood level of tryptophan in relation to other amino acids. This raised level leads to tryptophan being passed from the blood into the brain, where it then stimulates the production of another chemical called serotonin (otherwise known as 5HT). It is the raised level of 5HT that then decreases the appetite and lifts the misery associated with it.

For some years, medical scientists have been trying to find medication that would be of value in treating eating disorders such as bulimia. Much of this research revolved around anti-depressant drugs. Throughout the late 1970s and early 1980s, as more and more people with eating problems presented to mental health services, it was clear that many sufferers from bulimia were also depressed, and treatment with anti-depressant drugs was tried.

In general, these drugs did appear helpful. A review of twelve different clinical trials published in 1991 showed that in all but two studies, anti-depressants were more effective than placebos (dummy tablets) in the short-term treatment of normal-weight women with bulimia.[1] The long-term results were less certain and, in addition, a significant number of patients suffered from very considerable side-effects. The most common anti-depressant drugs that were used are known as the *tricyclic* anti-depressants, and their side-effects can include a dry mouth, constipation, sedation and dizziness. However, perhaps the most significant problem was that the vast majority of these anti-depressants lead to a slight increase in weight.[2] Hardly ideal in a problem such as bulimia.

However, a very promising breakthrough in the medical treatment of bulimia was the development of a group of drugs called SSRIs, or Selective Serotonin Re-uptake Inhibitors. Using this type of drug basically leads to an increase in the level of serotonin (5HT), and we have already seen how this can decrease appetite.

The Place of Prozac

Prozac is currently the only drug that is specifically licensed for the treatment of bulimia nervosa, used to reduce bingeing and purging. While Prozac is the name (brand name) by which most people know it, its chemical name is fluoxetine hydrochloride. In treating depression a dose of 20mg is usually given in tablet form in the morning; for bulimia a single daily morning dose of 60mg is recommended.

Prozac is an SSRI anti-depressant, and was first introduced in the late 1980s. Since then, there have been numerous trials looking at its use in bulimia nervosa. As an example, one major study in America and Canada looked at its use in 387 women who were treated in thirteen different specialist centres as out-patients.³ While this is only one of many such studies, it is a good example of the work that goes into such research.

The patients chosen for the trial were all over eighteen years of age, and were excluded if they were pregnant or breastfeeding, were significantly over or underweight, had serious medical or psychiatric illness, and if they had used other psychoactive drugs in the two weeks before the study, or other forms of therapy for bulimia (such as psychotherapy) in the month before the study started.

All patients in the study were given a placebo (usually a sugar tablet, used as a dummy treatment) for the first week. Those who had a 75 per cent improvement in this first week, or who had fewer than three bulimic episodes in this week, were excluded from the rest of the study. The remaining 387 patients were then randomly allocated to one of three groups. One group continued to receive the placebo. One group received 20mg Prozac each day, and the third received 60mg of Prozac. Neither the patients nor their therapists knew which group they were in.

They were seen regularly, and the study continued for eight weeks. The results were remarkable. In summary, 60mg of Prozac each day was much more effective than 20mg, which was in turn much better than the placebo.

Vomiting was reduced by 56 per cent in those on 60mg, by 29 per cent in those on 20mg, and 5 per cent in those on placebo. Binge-eating was also reduced, as were depression, carbohydrate craving, and abnormal eating behaviours and attitudes. All these results were judged from the patients' own diaries of binge-eating and purging. It was particularly interesting that the higher dose made such a difference. In studies of Prozac in depression this doesn't seem to happen, with 20mg being just as useful as higher doses.

What about side-effects?

There is no doubt that patients on Prozac in this study, as in most others, had more side-effects than those on placebo. The chief side-effects tend to be insomnia, nausea, tiredness and tremor. For instance ten patients on placebo complained that they couldn't sleep, compared to 23 per cent on 20mg Prozac, and 30 per cent on the 60mg dosage. Nausea occurred in 14 per cent, 20 per cent and 28 per cent respectively. Other side-effects have been reported with Prozac, though not in this particular study. These include such symptoms as sexual dysfunction (particularly a difficulty in reaching orgasm), rashes, loss of appetite with weight loss, and, very rarely, convulsions.

However, what was really significant was that patients on Prozac were no more likely to discontinue their treatment because they couldn't put up with the side-effects than those on placebos. It seems that the benefits far outweighed the problems. I have found that nausea is quite common with this drug, but warning patients about the problem seems to make it much more tolerable and it does gradually wear off. Incidentally, while most people do tolerate the higher 60mg morning daily dose every bit as well as the 20mg dose, not everyone can cope with it. In this case, taking just 20mg in the early evening can help considerably. This could be because the most common time for bingeing occurs in the evening, between six and twelve p.m. It could be that there is more drug in the bloodstream at this critical time, or it could be a psychological effect. Taking the drug at a high risk time just might be giving the potential binger more confidence.

In America there has been some controversy about the possibility of Prozac causing violent or suicidal behaviour. However, extensive medical research has not shown a genuine increase in this type of behaviour in people taking Prozac. A review in *Drug Safety News* in November 1993 confirmed the safety of this drug.[4]

One entirely different problem with Prozac can be its cost. At the time of writing, a daily dose of 60mg costs over £2 per day. A three-month course would be nearly two hundred pounds. The British government is putting pressure on doctors to reduce the cost of their prescribing, and it would be sad if the intensity of the pressure meant some patients did not get a drug that would help them very considerably.

Prozac usually takes about two weeks to have an anti-bulimic effect, although in a few patients this happens much sooner. Incidentally, it has a very prolonged action in the body. This means that if you are taking Prozac and you miss a dose, it isn't a problem. Missing the occasional dose, or having a dose that has not been fully absorbed (perhaps because of self-induced vomiting) isn't as dangerous as it would be with some other drugs. There will be enough drug still in your system to keep the effect going.

Is Prozac the answer to treating bulimia?

There can be no doubt that Prozac can be tremendously helpful in breaking the binge-purge cycle. However, we have already seen that there is far more to bulimia than simply a biochemical problem in part of the brain. Bio-chemistry is part of the problem, but it is only a part. There is as yet little evidence of the value of Prozac in long-term treatment, or what happens to sufferers from bulimia after the treatment has been discontinued.

What does seem very likely is that Prozac can buy time for the sufferer – a chance to escape from the cycle of bingeing and purging, and an opportunity to examine the whole psychological dimension of bulimia. It would seem sensible to continue it for some time after improvement has occurred. There aren't yet any long-term studies, but many experts have the impression that discontinuing treatment too early is likely to lead to a rapid return of symptoms. It seems far more valuable to continue it until the patient has begun to eat regular normal meals, and has begun to change her general attitudes towards eating, dieting and herself.

What does seem certain is that the length of time you are on the tablets is not important. Some people have taken them for two years and had a prompt relapse when the treatment was stopped. Others have been fine after just

170

a few weeks. It is the underlying bulimic attitudes that seem to matter. Prozac may not be the whole answer to bulimia, but it is an extremely useful step on the way.

A user's guide to Prozac

- Prozac may be prescribed under the name Prozac, or using the chemical name 'fluoxetine hydrochloride';
- the dose in bulimia is usually 60mg (three 20mg tablets) taken in the morning;
- the main side-effect is nausea. This usually improves with time;
- if nausea really is intolerable, try taking just 20mg in the early evening;
- Prozac may not work for up to two weeks. Be patient;
- if treatment is helpful, don't discontinue it until advised by your doctor;
- whilst Prozac is an anti-depressant, there is no evidence that it works in this way with bulimics. In studies on its effect in bulimia, improvement was not affected by any changes in depression. In other words, you don't just improve because you are less depressed;
- you will not gain weight. Weight loss, if any, tends to be very small;
- if you miss a dose, don't worry. Carry on as usual; and
- Prozac is definitely not the whole answer. Please read the next chapter on self-help.

Some sufferers from bulimia have found other forms of medication and medical care helpful. Homoeopathy, herbalism and acupuncture may have a place to play, and are generally very safe. However there have been no satisfactory controlled trials investigating how useful they can be, and until these have been carried out it is difficult to advise you which forms of complementary treatment might be the most helpful.

Helping Yourself: The Food Diary

If you were to ask a therapist to help you with your bulimia, the first thing that he or she would need to know would be details of how your bulimia affects you? When do you binge? Even more importantly, why do you binge? The fact that you are going to be your own therapist doesn't make this stage of understanding any less important.

You might think this is absurd. Of course you know when you binge! However, we have already seen how your image of yourself may not always be totally accurate. There's nothing unusual about that. Few of us have a good objective view of ourselves. It may well be the same when it comes to your eating problem. Perhaps it's not as bad as you think, or maybe it's worse. Until you really know and understand your own personal problem, you cannot start to tackle it.

The solution to this is simple and it really does work. You need to keep an accurate diary of your eating habits. Countless sufferers from bulimia have found that keeping an eating diary becomes an essential, fascinating and fundamental first step in saying goodbye to bulimia.

Many bulimics worry that this exercise may make them feel worse, by focusing their mind totally on the extent of the problem. However, if you really do want to change, then this is a step you must take. It is likely that you binge for a reason. Knowing every detail about your eating habits now will help to uncover some of the reasons and will give you a tremendous advantage when you are ready to change.

Keeping a Diary

Make yourself a simple diary in which to record your eating habits. The example on page 174 suggests a sample page. This is partially adapted, with permission, from the extremely effective diary system used for several years at the Royal Edinburgh Hospital in Scotland.

Ideally your food diary should be placed in a ring binder. It is important to have a separate page for each day. You can either draw out the plan yourself each day, or make photocopies of the outline given here. If you think photocopying is expensive, just work out the cost of your last binge!

An A4 binder may be too large, but you can carry the relevant pages throughout the day and insert them in the evening. Better still try making one to fit a personal organiser. Many stationery shops sell inexpensive versions which will be adequate, and you can easily adapt some of the pre-printed pages to become a bulimia diary.

Remember that my proposed outline is only a suggestion. If you want more space for your own comments, or to record other important aspects of your life, then please do so. This document is unique. It should be entirely personal to you, and reflect your needs and problems. However, it is far more than just a record. It is also an immensely powerful tool in helping you gain control over your eating.

The different columns should be used as follows:

- *Time*. Record this as accurately as you can. For instance, put 2.15 p.m., not just 'afternoon'.
- *Food or drink consumed*. Write down absolutely everything that passes your lips, and in as much detail as you can. Describe the food accurately, but don't weigh it and do not attempt to record its calorie content. From now on calories are forbidden. Don't

Your Eating Diary

Day:........................... Date: ....

Time	Food or drink consumed	Regrets?	Binge	Vomit	Laxative	How I feel at the moment

- The desire to starve myself today has been:

  |————————————————————————|

  Not at all   As strong as it possibly could be

- Today's urge to overeat has been:

  |————————————————————————|

  Not there at all   As strong as it possibly could be

- Today in general I have felt:

  |————————————————————————|

  Not emotionally upset at all   Extremely emotionally Upset

- What made me feel good today?

  |————————————————————————|

174

say 'crisps'; detail is important. Say 'two bags of Walker's crisps'. Be honest, accurate and try to avoid being obsessive.

- *Regrets?* Do you wish you hadn't eaten what you just ate? If so, put a tick in this column. You may have thought you had eaten too much. You may have regretted eating anything at all. Whatever the reason for your regret, record it here.
- *Binge.* If you consider that what you ate on this occasion was a binge, put a tick in this column.
- *Vomit* and *Laxative.* Record here whether you made yourself vomit, and any laxatives you took (with their quantity). If you have other ways of controlling your weight, such as exercise, you should adapt this column accordingly.
- *How I feel at the moment.* Use this column to record your mood at the time you ate. You may have felt angry about something, upset or worried. Record some detail – 'Upset because Simon didn't phone' or, 'Worried about exams' or, simply 'bored'. This might have been an occasion when you had to eat – in company with the family. Record how you felt about this. Don't think about what you write too much. Try to express your raw emotions. Remember, these are secret and personal.

The scales at the bottom of the page will give you a simple 'at a glance' view of your overall feelings on a given day. Later on they will also prove an invaluable guide to your progress – but don't worry about this yet.

Finally, the *'What made me feel good today?* question will allow you to list the things that helped you through the day. These will be different for everyone. It could be simple things like a long hot bath or a chat on the phone to a friend. It could be something active, like playing a favourite sport, or lazy, like snoozing in front of the television. You might have treated yourself to some new clothes, bought a record, springcleaned a room, gone to the cinema, done your hair differently. The potential for this list is endless, and it is invaluable. If you can identify the things that make you feel really good, then you might be able to use them when you would otherwise have turned to bingeing. The longer your list the better. Then you will have plenty of choices when the temptation to binge beckons.

Using the diary

There are a few useful rules about using a food diary.

- *Be totally honest.* You don't have to show your diary to anyone else. It is there so that you can learn to analyse and understand your behaviour. It is a totally personal and private document. If at any stage you do see a therapist, you may choose to share the contents of your diary, but don't let this thought make you censor your feelings, comments and recordings in any way. In addition, honesty is essential when it comes to monitoring how you are getting on with changing your bulimic behaviour.
- *If you are not doing as well as you hoped, still be totally honest.* How else will you know which things help, and which ones do not? It is terribly tempting to leave out a binge if you feel ashamed. It really is just as essential to record when things go badly as when things are going well. After all, an honest record may allow you to see why you are finding it difficult to change. Recording the truth accurately may actually disclose that parts of the day were far better than you feared.
- *Fill in the diary immediately after eating.* If you try to wait until the end of the day, you will find that you forget things, and it will be far less accurate.
- *Express your feelings freely.* Writing down your joys and fears, your worries and upsets, can be enormously therapeutic in itself. You may initially think that keeping a diary is tedious and boring. However, it will almost certainly turn into a fascinating document that will help you understand exactly how you tick.
- *Start keeping a diary as soon as you can.* Even if you don't feel that you will be able to change your behaviour just yet, it's helpful to have the diary as a record of your bulimic routines, and why and when

they are happening. Knowing how the problem really affects you is important and interesting. Your imagination may have been running wild.

Interpreting the diary

It is worth using your diary for at least a week before you even attempt to read anything into it. After a week, look back at the seven days and ask yourself a series of questions:

- What sort of events and situations trigger off my bingeing?
- How do I feel before I binge?
- How do I feel after a binge?
- In what way does bingeing seem to reward me?
- Are there times of the day or week when I'm more at risk of bingeing?
- What foods do I use to binge on?
- Do I eat regularly, or do I have spells when I hardly eat at all?
- What happens if I diet, or try to go without food?
- What makes me feel good?
- What do I eat that makes me feel good and in control?
- Do I find it difficult to express my true feelings?
- Does this make me more likely to binge?

Many sufferers from bulimia are simply unable to see the wood for the trees. They see themselves as weak, and their bulimia as disgusting. This book has shown that there is much more to it than that. Keeping a diary will allow you to see your problem in context.

Despite asking yourself these questions about your week's eating, you may still find it hard to understand what makes you binge. Here are a few more questions to think about:

- Am I being totally honest in my recordings?
- Do I binge when I am unhappy?
- Do I binge when I'm bored?
- Do I binge when I'm upset about myself?
- Do I binge when other people have upset me?

- Does bingeing make me feel calmer?
- Does bingeing make me feel in control?
- Does bingeing help me get at other people?
- Does bingeing give me sheer enjoyment?

If you purge, you need to ask yourself why. Do you purge for punishment, as an attempt to remove the calories you've binged, or because it makes you feel calmer?

At the end of each and every week, sit down and look at your charts. Ask yourself these questions, and try to understand the way that you work. If you later begin to share your diary with a therapist, he or she will stress that this is not a school test, with right and wrong answers. You will be encouraged to view each week's diary as an experiment in which you are trying to introduce certain changes to your behaviour and attitudes. But all experiments are scientific procedures, and you can learn just as much from a day or week that goes badly as from one that goes well. A bad day may teach you a great deal about yourself, and that in itself can be a major type of success.

For many sufferers from bulimia, keeping a diary can be the single most important step in learning to control their behaviour. It is not an optional extra. The rest of this book depends on it. And so does your future.

Helping Yourself: Normal Eating

Normal eating. What do those words mean to you? Quite possibly they will mean panic. Inevitable fatness. Uncontrollable weight gain. Understandably, most bulimia sufferers faced with the idea of returning to a normal eating pattern become nervous. Returning to a normal eating pattern means eating three regular meals, and a couple of snacks each day, but doing this instead of bingeing. Overall, if you eat a normal diet your over-all average food intake will almost certainly be less. You will not gain weight.

In Chapter 4 I explained how dieting makes you desperate for food, particularly the very foods that you are trying to avoid in the diet. Regular healthy eating will help prevent these powerful cravings. And the most important message of this chapter is:

NO MORE CALORIE-CONTROLLED DIETS

Calorie-controlled diets are part of the problem, not the solution. Setting fierce guidelines for yourself invites failure; and the feelings of failure simply go on to compound your feelings of worthlessness. Why complicate your life by giving yourself tough dietary rules that you may find impossible to keep?

Everyone finds it difficult to stick to an eating plan to begin with. Accept that you will make mistakes, but rather than descending into a panic attack when you make them, stop and think about the following points:

- everyone makes mistakes. You are no worse than anyone else;
- learn from the reasons why you binged. Look at your eating diary. Try to figure out what pushed you into this particular problem;
- a single lapse is not a disaster. It is simply one mistake. It need not turn the whole day into a write-off. You don't have to compound the problem by descending into a major binge; and
- try some basic relaxation techniques described in the next chapter. You do have more than one way of coping with stress and problems. You don't need to binge and purge.

There are some basic principles of normal eating that it is essential for you to understand. Like the eating diary, this list is adapted from one that has been successfully used by many bulimics at the Royal Edinburgh Hospital in Scotland.

Principles of Normal Eating

- Set aside some time daily to reflect on how you are coping. Some of your strategies may be working. Some may not.
- Plan your days ahead. Avoid both long periods of unstructured time and also over-booking. Don't put yourself under too much pressure.
- Use your eating diary to record absolutely everything that you eat.
- Try not to eat alone. It is far better to eat in company whenever you can.
- Do not do anything else while you eat, except social-ising. For instance, do not watch television. Do not read magazines or books. It is probably all right to listen to music or the radio, but you should still try to concentrate on the actual meal. This should apply both to binge and non-binge episodes.
- Plan to eat three meals each day, plus two snacks. Try to have these meals and snacks at pre-determined times. Plan your meals in detail so that you know exactly what and when you will be eating. In gen-

eral, you should try to keep one step ahead of your problem.

- Only have planned food in the house. Don't stock up too far ahead if you feel that you are at risk of buying too much food. Carry as little money as possible.
- From your diary, identify the times when you are most likely to overeat. Then plan alternative activities that are not compatible with eating. You might take a bath, meet friends, or go a walk. In your food diary there is a section for 'Things that made me feel good today'. Try one of these.
- When possible, avoid areas where food is kept. Try to keep out of the kitchen between meals and plan what you will do at the end of the meal. If really necessary, get out of the house straight away. The washing-up can wait!
- Don't weigh yourself more than once each week. If necessary, stop weighing altogether. Don't try to lose weight while you are trying to learn normal eating habits. Once you are eating normally, you may reduce weight if you want to by cutting down the quantities that you eat at each meal. Do not skip meals. Remember, gradual changes in weight are better for you and last far longer.
- If you find that you are always thinking about your shape and weight, this could possibly be because you are anxious or depressed. You tend to feel fat when things are not going well. Identify any particular current problems, and do something positive to solve or at least minimise them.
- Use exercise. Regular exercise increases your metabolic rate and helps to suppress your appetite – particularly your craving for carbohydrates.
- Be particularly aware in the days just before your period. Many women experience food cravings at this time.
- Avoid alcohol. This can increase your craving, and reduce your self-control.
- Set yourself limited and totally realistic goals. Work from hour to hour, rather than day to day. One failure does not justify a succession of failures. Note

your successes – however modest – in your diary. Every time you spend time eating normally you are reinforcing your new healthy eating habits.

In addition, it is worth remembering that many binges are effectively pre-planned. So, when shopping in your local supermarket, plan ahead. Don't stock up on extra supplies, to be stored in secret until they are needed. Buy food in small amounts. This may mean more trips to the shops, but it reduces potential binge foods, should the urge so take you. As an example, don't buy five litres of ice cream. Just buy half a litre at a time.

Yet again it is vital to reiterate the point that in order to overcome bulimia it is essential that you concentrate on normal eating and feeling well on your weight. Eating is not an indulgence to feel guilty about. It is a basic essential requirement of life. Of course, once you have gained control of your eating, then you will gradually be able to pay attention to your weight – if this is what you truly want. However, you will approach this issue slowly, avoiding the strict dieting that will inevitably bring back the cravings and the bingeing.

You won't be able to consider yourself free of bulimia until you achieve freedom from the pressures of dieting. There is no disguising the fact that being a non-dieter will be hard work, and won't be much fun to begin with. However, as you become better and better at being a non-dieter, the cravings to binge will begin to disappear. I cannot promise that they will go for ever, but they will ease very dramatically.

What do I do if I feel the need to binge?

Don't panic, and don't be surprised. For a long time now you have been dealing with your emotions by bingeing, so it's natural to be worried if the feelings come back. After all, coping with bulimia is stressful, and in the past your main way of dealing with stress has been bulimia.

But not any more. If you feel a binge coming on, employ delaying tactics. Do anything. For instance, the following may be appropriate for someone who spends most of their time at home. Your life may well be different, and it is important that it is personal to you. You could telephone a friend; go for a walk; polish the table; put on a record and sing along; run a hot bubble bath and pamper yourself; juggle; jog; dig the garden; prune the roses; do a jigsaw. The list is endless, and it's up to you to personalise it. Indeed, it is a good idea to have a written-out list of activities that you can do if the desire to binge comes on. In a crisis you can then work down your list. Try to choose more active pursuits rather than passive interests like watching television, and try to get away from the place where you do your bingeing. Don't include activities that you don't enjoy. If you enjoy vacuuming the carpet, then it can go on your list, but if you don't, then don't include it. Seeing it there will work as a disincentive. It should be as easy as possible to avoid bingeing.

Devote a page in your food diary to your list, but keep it up to date, and only use the activities which work, discarding the others.

Remember, you are stronger than the urge to binge. At the end of the day you can win. And every time that you avoid a binge will make the next time even easier. When you succeed, reward yourself. When you drew up your eating diary you produced a list of things that make you feel good. Use them. When you succeed, give yourself a treat – a magazine, a paperback, a T-shirt, a luxury coffee or cosmetics. This isn't being extravagant – just think how much bingeing used to cost you.

If you don't succeed, try not to despair. Your future isn't ruined. Get the bingeing and purging over with quickly, then start again. Back to your meal plan. No starving to compensate for the binge you just had. You know where that will lead to. Try to work out why the binge occurred, so that you can block it more effectively in future, and then write off the bad experience and start fresh.

In some of their excellent literature, the Eating Disorders Association (see page 216) makes many valuable recommendations, but one is particularly helpful at this time:

'Allow yourself to be real. Banish words like "should", "ought", "must", and "if only". Allow yourself to make mistakes and not be perfect, to live in the "grey" instead of the "black and white".'[1]

This really is essential. If you constantly expect yourself to be perfect, you are going to be disappointed. Be realistic. You will make mistakes, but that's okay. Put them behind you, and carry on.

Gaining control of your bulimia involves a number of steps:

- keeping an eating diary – to understand fully the pattern of your bulimia;
- learning about the stresses that cause you to binge;
- learning about the things that make you feel good;
- eating regularly – three meals a day, plus snacks, each and every day;
- accepting imperfection in yourself;
- sharing your problem – with friends, family, the EDA, your doctor, etc.;
- learning delaying tactics for when you feel the urge to binge;
- accepting that you have emotions, and allowing yourself to express them; and
- understanding the dreadful tyranny of the dieting industry, and beginning to accept that success and happiness do not automatically equal slimness.

Finally, you must accept that your problem has been brewing for a long time. It will not disappear overnight. However, think of every positive step as part of the way forward. Each time you manage to resist a binge, and every day that you eat normally is a very real achievement. Value yourself. I have talked a great deal in this book about vicious cycles, but the opposite, more benign cycles, apply as well. Every time that you succeed at something, this will help your self-confidence. Self-esteem can be built by success, just as it can be knocked down by problems. Knowing that you are far from being alone in your bulimia will help you feel less guilty and ashamed.

The self-help techniques suggested in these last two

chapters should make a real difference to your life. However, there is no doubt that some people with bulimia do have a problem that is simply too severe for self-help.

If this is the case, the next step might be the Eating Disorders Association's excellent 'Supported Self-Help Programme', which uses similar techniques but with the support of an EDA telephone counsellor, and regular weigh-ins by your doctor. Alternatively, your doctor will be able to put you in contact with specialised local help. If self-help is not the answer for you, don't give up. Plenty more help is available.

The next chapter looks at some of the other strategies that you can use to help you cope with the stresses of everyday life, and to begin to care for your body.

21

Looking After Yourself

Throughout this book I have stressed that bulimia cannot be tackled as an isolated problem. Your bulimia probably occurred as a result of a combination of factors – some personal, some biochemical and others the product of social pressures.

However well you have tackled the problem of binge eating and your other bulimic symptoms, you are still living in a world of frustrations, pressures, pleasure and pain. You cannot assume that you will never ever again be tempted by bulimia. You need to be aware that the ever-present pleasure of food may combine with a period of very major stress, and you may find the pressure to binge again surprisingly strong.

So now is the time to look at alternative ways of caring for yourself. Accept the fact that you will face stress throughout your life and look for ways to handle it. Learn how to use food as a friend, rather than a potential enemy. In addition, you will need to wean yourself from laxatives and diuretics, and take care of some of the other physical problems that bulimia may have caused for you.

Coping with Stress

By using some of the diary-keeping techniques that I have already described, you have gone a long way towards beginning to conquer the stresses in your life. Recognising the enemy is half the battle. Indeed, the act of finding the source of your stress is frequently relief enough in itself. It may be that you have been comparing yourself unfavourably with friends, relatives and those around you, while forgetting that they may be as stressed as you are. Your poor self-esteem may have made you assume that you are simply less competent than everyone else. Indeed, it is possible that you have blamed one particular cause while the actual trigger for your stress has been something quite different.

However, there are still going to be occasions when all the self-understanding in the world is not going to be enough to take all your stress away. Understanding the causes better may well turn down the volume of stress, but it may not turn it off completely. It is for these occasions that this section is intended. This is general advice that can help anyone, but it is important to diagnose the causes of your individual stress in order to best treat it.

Relaxation and fitness

The first and golden rule of relaxation is that it does not mean that you simply do nothing. Of course, there is nothing wrong with the occasional mindless night watching television, but it is not enough to cure stress. Too little stress can actually be as harmful as too much. There is little doubt that the best way to unwind is to do something that requires your full attention, but is a different stress altogether from the pressures that normally hound you.

For example, I have found the perfect cure for the stresses that affect me during the hectic winter period. Few doctors enjoy the winter. Colds, flu and one virus after another leads to a busy lifestyle becoming doubly so. However, my perfect relaxation has turned out to be skiing. Nothing else that I have ever done has relaxed me so completely, and the reason is simple. It requires complete and total mental concentration, and results in physical exhaustion. I am completely unable to think or worry about what is happening back in the practice while I am trying to stay upright on a snow-covered mountainside. Lying on a beach, or watching the television, might seem more relaxing, but for many people it is simply not enough. The mind can keep drifting back to the pressures and problems of everyday life.

Now, the last thing that I am suggesting is that you go skiing every time you feel stressed but I do recommend that you find regular physical activity that occupies both your mind and your body. Stretch, occupy and relax your mind by learning a musical instrument, reading, or taking up a hobby. Similarly, choose some form of regular exercise that you can enjoy and which keeps your body agile and active. From a point of view of health, and preventing heart attacks, it has been shown that three twenty-minute episodes of exercise every week can be enormously beneficial and can make an enormous difference to the way you feel both physically and mentally. People often say that they don't have time for exercise, but as a rule of thumb, you always make time for the things that are important to you. Finding exercise that you enjoy will be a pleasure to fit into a busy schedule.

The vital rules about exercise are to take it gently to begin with, and to do it regularly. The stressed person who takes no exercise for months on end and then suddenly has a highly aggressive game of squash is probably doing him or herself more harm than good. And, there is more to exercise as a treatment for stress than just a pleasant feeling of tiredness and self-righteousness. The fitter you are physically, the better able you are to cope with stress. It is something we all have experienced. For example, when you have a cold, minor problems are likely to cause you far more aggravation than when you feel fit and well.

However, there is yet another side to exercise and stress. Stress has very marked physical effects on the body, and in particular prepares us for 'fight or flight'. The muscles get tensed up ready for action. The heart pounds. The body prepares for exercise. Well, what better way to help the body than to give it the exercise it is preparing for?

Finally, too much stress tends to affect your self-image and self-confidence. Stressed people often feel very negative about themselves. Feeling physically fit often does the very opposite: the fit person stands tall, and tends to feel much more confident. Dealing with stress should be an important part of each day.

Learning Relaxation Techniques

However important physical fitness may be, you will still probably need to learn ways of dealing with major stresses in an emergency, or when you simply feel yourself getting unbearably tense. Swallowing tranquillisers is not the answer, but learning proper relaxation techniques may well be. And your body may certainly need help. I have already mentioned the profound physical effects that stress can have on the body – the heart races, the mouth goes dry, muscles go tense, legs feel like jelly, and the poor sufferer feels a desperate need to go to the toilet.

Not surprisingly, a truly relaxed person feels almost the complete opposite of this:

- the heart slows down;
- breathing becomes slower and regular;
- blood pressure falls;
- muscles become less tense;
- the person feels very calm; and
- most bodily activities appear to slow down.

Until the 1960s most psychologists agreed that 'switching off' was an acceptable way of relaxing. However, it is now well established that there is more to true relaxation than simply resting. It is a genuine skill, a technique that can be worked at and improved like any other. People who master the skills required can often calm themselves rapidly and dramatically. Some people can relax naturally. They can sit down in a chair and doze contentedly for a few minutes, then wake refreshed and ready to do battle with all that life flings at them. Others find it very much harder. You might try pampering yourself in a long hot bath, but this is of course entirely useless if you spend the whole time thinking about the jobs that need doing when you get out.

So how can you learn to relax more effectively? There are a number of tips which can help:

- try exercising before you relax. Many people find it easier to switch into relaxation after some physical exercise;
- alternatively, try relaxing after a warm but not hot bath;
- try and choose a regular routine time to relax;
- try some simple relaxation exercises (see below); and
- try yoga or meditation, which can be enormously beneficial. You should be able to find classes.

There is one particular form of relaxation which I have found particularly effective. This involves a simple exercise, which you will need to practise regularly to get the full benefit. Practise it when you feel calm and in control. Later you'll find it that much easier to use when you feel stressed, tense and angry. Once you have mastered the art of relaxation you will be able to use it at will, but if you have not practised beforehand it is much harder to achieve a relaxed state.

For this particular exercise you need to wear loose clothing and lie flat on your back. Start by screwing up your face muscles as tightly as you can, and then let them relax. Work through all the face muscles in turn: frowning to tense the forehead and then relaxing; screwing up the eyes and then relaxing; clenching the jaw and then letting it fall loose.

When you have relaxed the face, next lift up your head and let it fall gently back. Next relax your shoulders. Start by pressing them down and then let them go loose. The arms and fingers are next, and the technique is similar. Hold them out to the side and make them as taut as you can, and then relax them completely. Finally lift each leg into the air for thirty seconds, making the muscles as tight as you can, then let them go limp, and drop back down.

When you are practising, relax the legs, arms, neck, forehead, eyes and jaw one after the other for about ten minutes. Then lie still and relaxed for a little while, enjoying the feeling of loosened muscles.

Laboratory tests have shown that a spell of concentrated relaxation like this can be more beneficial than a standard dose of a tranquilliser drug, with no side-effects. And you are able to use the technique at will. You will soon be able to use this form of relaxation at a few moments' notice, and will be able to get back in control of your stress rapidly and safely.

Some people find that slow, deep breathing can be extremely helpful as a form of relaxation. To practise this, you simply need to breathe slowly and deeply for a minute at about half the speed you normally breathe. If you feel dizzy, stop. You are probably going too fast. If you can combine this kind of breathing with muscular relaxation then you will get even greater benefit.

The Simple Things of Life

In all this discussion of powerful and tested techniques for helping you to relax, please don't forget the simple relaxations as well. Laughter, for instance, can be an enormously powerful reliever of stress. Scientific tests have shown that it increases the level of endorphins in the body. These are the natural morphine-like substances that can ease pain and stress. And you always knew you felt better after a good laugh.

Don't forget music, books, television and pets. It has been proved that blood pressure falls when owners cuddle up and fuss their pets.

Weaning Yourself off Laxatives and Diuretics

In Chapter 4 we discussed how useless laxatives and diuretics actually are in helping you control your weight. However, since you have probably become used to taking them, stopping them suddenly is hopeless. You will almost certainly develop a rebound water retention that will make you feel excessively bloated and uncomfortable, and may put you under irresistible pressure to begin using them again.

Instead, make a chart that will help you to reduce them by a regular set amount. As an example, if you currently take twenty laxatives each day, reduce by one each day so that over the next three weeks you will have stopped them in a series of tiny, almost imperceptible steps. If you need help in drawing up a withdrawal regime, ask for your doctor's help.

And when you have stopped using them, never use them again. If you decide to save a few to use 'in an emergency' then you are still dependent on them. Breaking the laxative habit is worthwhile in the long run. When you have weaned yourself, why not flush your remaining supplies down the toilet and cut out the middle man? As you reduce your laxatives intake, it is sensible to drink at least six glasses of water each day, and to avoid a high-fibre diet as this can cause abdominal cramps and bloating at this stage. When you have finished taking laxatives altogether, then slowly and very gradually re-introduce fibre into your diet. It is likely to be several months before your bowel function returns completely to normal, and so patience is absolutely essential.

Most people these days have a pretty good idea of what foods contain the most fibre, so a low-fibre diet would take you in the opposite direction. During the low-fibre stage, before you slowly reintroduce fibre into your diet, try:

- lean meat and poultry or fish;
- white bread, but not wholemeal;
- bananas and cooked fruit, but not raw fruit with their seeds or skins;
- spaghetti and macaroni, but not bran or brown rice; and
- cooked or lightly steamed vegetables, but not raw vegetables with their skins.

Dental Health

Repeated episodes of self-induced vomiting can cause considerable damage to tooth enamel. Many bulimics make the problem worse by brushing their teeth after they have vomited to try to get rid of the smell. If you are still vomiting occasionally, avoid brushing. Instead, rinse your mouth over and over again with water and try not to eat for the next couple of hours.

Be honest with your dentist. If you explain the cause of your problems and ask for guidance and help, you will do far better than if you make up some other far-fetched explanation for the state of decay in your mouth.

Healthy Eating

In the last chapter I have stressed many of the important rules of normal eating. However, there are a few basic guidelines to eating healthily which are worth bearing in mind. This book is not the place to discuss all the modern views on a healthy diet at any length; however, I will briefly summarise the most important aspects.

The main rules of healthy eating that everyone should follow are:

Eat less fat. There is a very close link between certain types of dietary fat and heart disease. By following these few simple tips you can successfully and painlessly reduce the amount of fat in your diet:

- grill, don't fry;
- cut the visible fat off meat before you cook it;
- reduce the amount of full-fat cheese, butter and cream that you eat;
- change from full-cream milk to fresh skimmed or semi-skimmed; and
- eat less red meat, and more fish and poultry.

Eat more fibre. This definitely does not mean that you need to go out and buy fibre tablets or special supplements. It is far easier and healthier for you and your family to eat more fresh fruit and vegetables, more potatoes and other root crops, and more peas and beans. Eat more bread too – wholemeal is best – and pasta is excellent, too.

Eat less sugar. We each eat about 40kg of sugar each year. That is worth 150,000 calories a year, or 410 calories a day. However, most of this is hidden in processed and tinned foods, cakes, biscuits and cereals. You may have thrown away your sugar bowl and still have a high sugar intake. It is worth cutting down on all foods with a high sugar content, and certainly avoid adding sugar to drinks. It may take you some time to lose your sweet tooth, but it's well worth it.

Eat less salt. The amount of salt we actually need is tiny, so cutting back can do no harm. As most of us get around a third of our salt from that added in cooking or at the table, then throwing away the salt cellar may be all you need to do. Foods with a high salt content also include salted peanuts, crisps, sauces, tinned vegetables and tinned soups, although tinned vegetables with no added salt are now on the market.

But remember, above all else, that food is for enjoying. Choose a mixture of foods, and every day try to choose at least one food from the following food groups:

- bread, cereals, pasta and rice;
- fruit and vegetables, including potatoes;
- milk, cheese and yoghurt; and
- meat, fish, pulses, eggs and nuts.

You may be surprised to see bread, potatoes and other carbohydrates in this list. These aren't an optional extra. They are essential, if possible at every meal.

In this chapter and the last you have learnt many of the basic rules of healthy and normal eating. If you do want to lose weight, stick to these guidelines and take it gently. And it really is essential that you keep away from meal supplements. The goal is healthy normal eating. No one could pretend that substituting a meal with a specially formulated milkshake, bar or tablet constitutes 'normal' eating.

Gynaecological Problems

Many women with bulimia have problems with their periods. Periods often become very infrequent or even stop altogether. However this is a temporary problem, as dealing with the bulimia usually results in your cycle returning to normal. It is also important to realise that bulimia does not make you sterile. Indeed, even if your periods have stopped, it is still important to use contraceptive precautions as pregnancy may occasionally occur in women recovering from bulimia whose periods have not yet started.

If you are still actively bulimic, the oral contraceptive pill is probably not ideal for you. Vomiting or diarrhoea can affect the absorption of the Pill, so self-induced vomiting or laxative abuse can result in the Pill being unreliable. If you are on the Pill, or are considering starting it, do ensure that you take it at a time when your bulimic activities are unlikely to interfere with its absorption. Otherwise, discuss the question of contraception with your doctor, or a counsellor at a family planning clinic. If you use the contraceptive cap (diaphragm) and either lose or gain a significant amount of weight – half a stone or more – go and check that it still fits correctly. A good fit is essential to its efficiency.

It is obviously preferable to avoid pregnancy until you have sorted out your bulimia. However, if you do become pregnant, either deliberately or accidentally, there is really very little evidence that bulimia affects the growth of the baby in any way. People with bulimia who become pregnant often become so anxious about the possible effects of the bulimia on their unborn baby that their bulimia gets worse and worse. So, if this applies to you, stop worrying. Your baby will take the nourishment that he or she needs. Any deficiencies of iron, calcium or vitamins may affect you, but they won't affect your baby. Remember that repeated vomiting can cause electrolyte disturbances, and diuretics and laxatives might also have a damaging effect on the foetus. There is also plenty of evidence that a supplement of folic acid taken prior to becoming pregnant does significantly reduce the risk of spina bifida. Your pharmacist, doctor, or local midwife would be happy to give advice on this. A multivitamin supplement might also be valuable for women who have recently recovered from bulimia.

Nevertheless, if you are considering having a baby, work through your bulimia first. Emotionally and physically you will be in far better shape, not only for your pregnancy, but also for providing your baby for a happy, healthy and relaxed environment to grow up in.

22

Bulimia in Family and Friends

Discovering that someone that you care about suffers from bulimia can be dreadfully upsetting. You thought you knew them, and now this has come to light. If the person with bulimia is a member of your family, your concern may be mingled with feelings of guilt. If you are a parent, you may be wondering if the problem is your fault. You need to know what to do now, how best to help, what you should say and what you should avoid saying.

Bulimia is not a 'slimming' disease. It is a sign of more deeply rooted problems, and I do believe that it is important that you understand them. You need to understand bulimia in some detail, so this chapter should be read in conjunction with the rest of the book.

One of the most important concepts to understand is covered in detail in the first part of the book: you have to consider the actual way that the bulimic person behaves, the way she feels about herself and her world, and the way she handles her emotions. People with bulimia use bingeing and purging to help themselves handle difficult emotions. Perhaps you do something different – maybe you shout, argue or cry, or maybe you smoke, exercise or drink. All of these can help you deal with your emotions and feelings. People with bulimia find it very hard to express many emotions, and use the distraction of the bulimia to help them forget how bad they feel.

How Can I Help?

Learn about the condition. The more you understand bulimia, its complexity and causes, the better. Reading this book is an excellent first step. The whole problem is frequently incomprehensible to non-bulimics, which is the reason I have quoted so many case histories in this book. If you can begin to understand the reasons why someone with bulimia behaves the way she does, it will become much less frightening and puzzling.

Give her plenty of time. Be as supportive as you can. Listen when she wants to talk. But do not try and take over and control her life. That is the last thing that she needs. The self-help techniques discussed in Chapters 19 and 20 depend on the individual taking responsibility for her own emotions and actions. People with bulimia use it to help them feel more in control. You must be as supportive as you can without taking over. Offer help, but don't insist that it is accepted.

Don't feel upset if the person with bulimia wants to use an outside therapist. You may simply be too close to be able to be objective. I know that I am completely unable to be a doctor to my own family. The bulimic really does need an impartial, outside uninvolved person to whom she can talk.

Don't hesitate to seek help for yourself, if you feel you need it. You may find the whole subject terribly distressing. Talk to your doctor about your own feelings, or contact the Eating Disorders Association (see page 216). It can be desperately upsetting watching someone that you love hurt herself. Look after yourself, too.

What if she hasn't owned up yet?

It may be that you have discovered that your loved one is bulimic, but that this discovery is not yet in the open. I would suggest that you don't begin by asking her about eating or weight. She is apt to be defensive, and probably frightened of the idea of treatment. Many people believe that treatment will inevitably result in their being forced to eat much more, with subsequent weight gain, and they are also very frightened of failing. In addition, she may find it easy to deny that eating is a problem.

Instead, try to encourage her to talk about the way she feels. You could comment that she looks under the weather, or seems tense or depressed. You might be able to comment on any other symptoms that have become apparent, like sleep problems. Don't push it. Don't be aggressive. One of the techniques that I find most useful as a doctor is simply to say, 'You don't seem very happy', and then wait. The fears and worries flood out.

If she agrees that she does have a problem, then suggest she seeks professional help. If she agrees, phone and make an appointment right away, before she has a chance to change her mind. If she refuses, leave it. Try again another day. Don't get angry and don't try and force her. The chances are that your anger will make her more tense and fearful, and the problem then deepens rather than eases. Remember, if she is bulimic, she knows it. Any denial is part of her reluctance to admit openly that she is less than perfect. If nothing else, just let her know that you are happy to talk if she ever wants to.

However, I am not suggesting that you pretend that there is nothing wrong. Let her know that you realise what is happening, that she is bulimic, that you feel upset seeing her so miserable, and that you are happy to lend support and encouragement whenever she is ready.

What if she refuses treatment?

If she does accept that she has a problem, but refuses to see anyone for treatment, then the most likely reason is that she is afraid of what the treatment will involve. She may have dreadful images of being force-fed, or being judged or criticised. She may be worried about being labelled as mentally ill, or being a failure.

The simplest answer to this is to encourage her to read this book. I have tried to explain the various treatment techniques in a straightforward way, and when she discovers that they will not be quite as dreadful as she feared, then she will be far more likely to accept help.

Finally, if she won't consult anyone face to face, she might be prepared to accept the relative anonymity of a telephone discussion with an Eating Disorders Association counsellor.

What do I do when she is in treatment?

Many parents and friends do not know what to do while the bulimic person is being treated. Should they ask how the treatment is going? Should they comment about how she seems to be getting on?

There is one simple answer. Ask her if she wants to talk about it. Some people feel deeply hurt that their parents and friends don't discuss matters with them. Others feel that discussion means that the family and friends are trying to take over.

If she threatens to drop out of therapy, this may be because she feels she is failing. Don't forget that many bulimia sufferers tend to be impatient and impulsive. She may simply feel she is not improving as rapidly as she would like. If this is the case, remind her that the treatment can take every bit as long as the duration of the illness itself. Stress that you don't mind the length of time it takes. She may also be afraid of what is happening, afraid of talking about some of the emotions that are coming near to the surface. She may be worried that she will lose control, and she may even be afraid of the consequences of being well.

If this is the case, remind her that being well does not mean that she has to be or do anything that she doesn't want. She doesn't have to change in any other way. Part of being well is being in control of herself and her future. That can be quite a frightening thought.

If she stops her treatment, but won't talk to you about it, again I would suggest a very laidback approach. Say that you are available to talk if she wants, and that you are concerned, but leave it at that. Don't be judgemental.

There are a few other hints to take into consideration while she is in treatment. Some of these may not be easy, but I would urge you to follow them if you possibly can:

- allow her as much control as possible with regard to choosing meals, shopping, etc.;
- make mealtimes as relaxing as possible. Don't discuss problems over meals. Choose another time for this;
- try not to comment about her shape and weight. These are infinitely less important than healthy eating. If she asks about her weight, do remember that at the beginning of a treatment plan, many people temporarily gain a small amount. Remind her of this, and encourage her to stick with the plan;
- try not to watch her while she is eating. Difficult, but essential if she is to lower the emotional aspects of eating;
- don't try to catch her out. Don't listen at the bathroom door to see if she is vomiting. She needs to learn trust. If she finds out, the anger and resentment will make things much worse;
- keeping the foods she binges on out of the house will not prevent her from bingeing. Ask her if she would prefer these foods to be kept out, but don't forget the rest of the family has rights and preferences, too; and
- if you find that she has binged, say so – but not critically.

At all times try and remember that the best way of developing trust and friendship is by being honest and open. Put yourself in her shoes and remember it is all going to take time. It will be worth it.

Summary

- Don't feel guilty.
- Learn as much as you possibly can about bulimia.
- Be supportive, but don't try to take over.
- Don't try and force the person with bulimia into treatment, but be available and encouraging when she chooses.
- Find out what she wants.
- Don't let her bulimia take over your life. You matter

too. If you want her to learn to be open and to express emotions, then you are certainly entitled to do this as well.

And is it all worth it? Helen wrote me a long letter about her bulimia and admitted that, 'I became dreadfully impatient with people, and a real pain to be around. I was tearful, impulsive and miserable. The thing that most helped me was knowing that I was not alone in the world, my family, and my friends, who had unending support and patience, and who showed me nothing but kindness.'

Conclusion

Bulimia nervosa can be a devastating experience for those who suffer from it, and for their loved ones. However, the much greater openness about the condition in the past couple of years, particularly highlighted by the Princess of Wales' highly publicised speech on the topic, means that no one now needs to feel alone. Family doctors are receiving more and more information about the topic. Self-help groups, despite often struggling for funds, provide a vitally important service. An increasing amount of research is being carried out to help pinpoint the best treatments, psychological and medical.

In the long run, we need to find a way to prevent bulimia. Better understanding will be the key to this, but dramatic social changes are also essential. The tyranny of thinness in fashion has to change. This may not be as hopeless a possibility as it might seem. Take another aspect of our appearance that has health implications – sun-tans and skin cancer. For years, tanned skin had been equated with health, attractiveness and sexuality. Increased awareness of the very real risks of skin cancer means that more and more people are keeping out of the direct sun. Good sense is winning. The health risks of bulimia are every bit as great as the risks of skin cancer. Maybe, with education and time, attitudes will gradually change.

The outlook for the vast majority of people with bulimia, who work through a treatment plan like the ones I have discussed in this book, is extremely good. Eighty per cent of people with bulimia show improvement after a five-year period. However, early presentation can make all the difference. The best outcomes seem to occur with sufferers who are less than twenty years old when they first seek help, and with a history of less than five years of binge eating. Seeking help early means a better result, and increased publicity and education about the condition should mean that more people seek help much sooner.

Can you ever be completely free of bulimia? This seemingly simple question is remarkably difficult to answer, as it all depends on how you would define total cure. Many people who have never been bulimic comfort eat on occasions when they are under stress. If you ever do this in the future will you consider that you have failed and that the bulimia has returned? While many people who recover from bulimia are able to eat perfectly normally, without any worries about their weight and shape, there are others who remain occasionally at risk of bingeing, especially if they are under great stress.

It is essential that your goals for recovery are personal to you, are sensible and are realistic. You also need to be aware that a setback is not a disaster. As I have stressed over and over again, bulimia is not in charge of you. It is not a monster threatening to take you over if you let your guard slip. If, after having eaten normally with no binges for many months, you then slip up and binge, it does not mean that the bulimia has won. Put it behind you, and carry on. Every single one of us has weaknesses, and you are no different. Accepting your normality in this way is an essential part of your recovery.

So take your recovery at your own pace; your life will gradually improve. Your future has such great potential. You now have the opportunity to put your bulimia behind you. It won't be easy, but it will be worthwhile.

The last words should come from someone who has had bulimia. Louise had suffered from bulimia for years. She wrote to me at length about her experiences of bingeing and purging. After one day collapsing in the toilet, she said:

I don't know what happened. I had taken so many laxatives, I had just lost count. My mum heard me hit my head as I fell off the toilet – it was the first she knew of it all. She called for my doctor, and shortly afterwards I started at an eating disorders group.

It was good. I found that others felt like I did too. Astonishing. The group followed a ten-week plan of weekly meetings, and followed an eating plan. After the first week or so I didn't particularly enjoy it, but something must have worked. Since about the eighth week of treatment I have never binged again, and that was three years ago.

Now I never have the urge to binge. I actually let myself eat chocolate, and I never feel guilty. I experience hunger pangs and don't eat so much that I feel bloated. My weight has remained steady at nine and a half stone and I'm happy with my body, I accept the shape that I am.

What is most wonderful is that I now feel all kinds of emotions that I never had before. I've stopped trying to keep them in. I really do seem to be a very different person, happily married to a man who knows all about my past bulimia and has accepted me the way that I am. I'm writing to you because I am so anxious to help others, and to let them know that recovery is possible.

References

Chapter 1

1. Edwards-Hewitt, T., Gray, J.J., 'The Prevalence of Disordered Eating Attitudes and Behaviours in Black-American and White-American College Women: Ethnic, Regional, Class, and Media Differences'. *Eating Disorders Review*, 1993, 1, (1) 41–54.

2. Bruch, Hilde, *Eating Disorders*. London: Routledge & Kegan Paul, 1974.

3. Russell, G.F., 'Bulimia Nervosa: An Ominous Variant of Anorexia Nervosa'. *Psychological Medicine*, 1979, 9, 429–448.

4. *Daily Star*, 28 April 1993, p. 7.

5. Carter, R., 'Eating Disorders – What We Know Now'. *She*, September 1993, 74–76.

6. *Empire*, June 1993, p. 50.

7. Redgrave, L., *Diet for Life*. London: Penguin Books, 1993.

8. American Psychiatric Association: *Diagnostic and Statistical Manual of Mental Disorders* (3rd Ed.). Washington: 1980, p. 70.

9. American Psychiatric Association: *Diagnostic and Statistical Manual of Mental Disorders* (3rd Ed. Rev.). Washington: 1987, p. 67.

10. Parkin, J.R., Eagles, J.M., 'Blood-Letting in Bulimia Nervosa'. *British Journal of Psychiatry*, 1993, 162, 246–248.

Chapter 2

1. Fairburn, C.G., Beglin, S.J., 'Studies of the Epidemiology of Bulimia Nervosa'. *American Journal of Psychiatry*, 1990, 147, 401–408.
2. Roberts and Schoelkopf, 'Eating, Sleeping and Elimination Practices in a Group of 2½-year-old Children'. *American Journal of Diseases of Childhood*, 82, 121–152.
3. Newson, J., Newson, E., 'Four Years Old in an Urban Community'. London: Pelican Books, 1970.
4. Bruch, Hilde, *Eating Disorders*. London: Routledge & Kegan Paul, 1974.
5. Schmidt, U., Hodes, M., Treasure, J., 'Early onset Bulimia Nervosa: Who Is at Risk? A Retrospective Case-control Study'. *Psychological Medicine*, 1992, 22, (3) 623–628.
6. Lacey, J.H., 'Bulimia Nervosa, Binge-eating and Psychogenic Vomiting: A Controlled Treatment Study and Long-term Outcome'. *British Medical Journal*, 1983, 286, 1609–1613.
7. Lacey, J.H., Mourelli, E., 'Bulimic Alcoholics: Some Features of a Clinical Sub-group'. *British Journal of Addiction*, 1986, 81, 389–393.
8. Lacey, J.H. Read, T.R.C., 'Multi-impulsive Bulimia: Description of an In-patient Eclectic Treatment Programme and a Pilot Follow-up Study of its Efficacy', *Eating Disorders Review*, 1993, 1, 22–31.

Chapter 3

1. Johnson, C.L., et al, 'Bulimia: A Descriptive Survey of 316 Cases'. *International Journal of Eating Disorders*, 1982, 2, 3–15.
2. Haslam, D., 'An Approach to Psychosocial Problems'. *The Physician*, July 1984, 32–33.
3. Haslam, D., *Parent Stress*. London: Futura Books, 1989.

Chapter 4

1. Johnson, C.L., et al, 'Bulimia: A Descriptive Survey of 316 Cases'. *International Journal of Eating Disorders*, 1982, 2, 3–15.
2. Blackburn, G.L, et al, 'Weight Cycling: The Experience of Human Dieters'. *American Journal of Clinical Nutrition*,

1989, 49, 1105–1109.

3. Folkins, C.H., Sime, W.E., 'Physical Fitness Training and Mental Health'. *American Psychologist*, 1986, 36, 373–389.

4. Chow, R., Harrison, J.E., Notarius, C., 'Effect of Two Randomised Exercise Programmes on Bone Mass of Healthy Post-menopausal Women'. *British Medical Journal*, 1987, 295, 1441–1044.

5. Stern, J.S., 'Is Obesity a Disease of Inactivity?' *Eating and Its Disorders*, Ed A.J. Stunkard and E. Stellar. New York: Raven Press, 1984.

6. Anon., 'Trapped in a vicious circle'. *Monitor Weekly*, 14 July 1993.

7. Eyton, A., *The F-Plan Diet*. London: Penguin Books, 1982.

Chapter 5

1. Royal College of General Practitioners, 'The Future General Practitioner – *Learning & Teaching*'. *British Medical Journal*, 1972.

2. Dunne, F., Schipperheijn, J., Feeney, S., 'Eating Disorders and the Cardiovascular System'. *Psychiatry in Practice*, Autumn 1993, 22–23.

3. Broberg, D.J., Bernstein, I.L., 'Preabsorptive Insulin Release in Bulimic Women and Chronic Dieters'. *Appetite*, 1989, 13, 161–169.

4. Schweiger, U., et al, 'Altered Insulin Response to a Balanced Test Meal in Bulimic Patients'. *International Journal of Eating Disorders*, 1987, 6, 551–556.

5. Ravussin, E., et al, 'Reduced Rate of Energy Expenditure as a Risk Factor for Body Weight Gain', *New England Journal of Medicine*, 1988, 318, 467–472.

6. Elliot, D.L., Goldberg, L., Kuehl, K.S., Bennett, W.M., 'Sustained Depression of the Resting Metabolic Rate after Massive Weight Loss'. *American Journal of Clinical Nutrition*, 1989, 49, 93–96.

7. Poehlman, E.T., Horton, E.S., 'The Impact of Food Intake and Exercise on Energy Expenditure', *Nutrition Reviews*, 1989, 47, 129–137.

Chapter 6

1. Russell, G.F., 'Bulimia Nervosa: An Ominous Variant of

Anorexia Nervosa'. *Psychological Medicine*, 1979, 9, 429–448.

2.   Orbach, S., *Hunger Strike*. London: Penguin Books, 1993.
3.   Pope, H.G., Hudson, J.L., Yurgelun-Todd, D., Hudson, M.S., 'Prevalence of Anorexia Nervosa and Bulimia in Three Student Populations'. *International Journal of Eating Disorders*, 1984, 3, (3), 45–51.
4.   Katzman, M.A., Wolchik, S.A., Braver, S.L., 'The Prevalence of Frequent Binge-eating and Bulimia in a Non-clinical College Sample'. *International Journal of Eating Disorders*, 1984, 3, (3), 53–61.
5.   Fairburn, C.G., Beglin, S.J., 'Studies of the Epidemiology of Bulimia Nervosa'. *American Journal of Psychiatry*, 1990, 147, 401–408.
6.   Johnson, C.L., Tobin, D.L., Lipkin, J., 'Epidemiologic Changes in Bulimia Behaviour Among Female Adolescents over a 5-Year Period'. *International Journal of Eating Disorders*, 1991.
7.   Pyle, R.L., et al, 'The Increasing Prevalence of Bulimia in Freshman College Students'. *International Journal of Eating Disorders*, 1986, 5, 563–568.
8.   Carlat, D.J., Camargo, C.A., 'Review of Bulimia Nervosa in Males'. *American Journal of Psychiatry*, 1991, 148, 831–843.
9.   Striegel-Moore, R.H., Silberstein, L.R., Frensch, P., Rodin, J., *International Journal of Eating Disorders*, 1989, 8, (5), 499–509.
10.   Smith, J.E., Krejci, J., *International Journal of Eating Disorders*, 1991, 10, (2), 179–186.
11.   Halmi, K.A., Falk, J.R., Schwartz, E., 'Binge-Eating and Vomiting: A Survey of a College Population'. *Psychological Medicine*, 1981, 11, 697–706.
12.   Klemchuk, H.P., Hutchinson, C.B., Frank, R.I., 'Body Dissatisfaction and Eating-related Problems on the College Campus: Usefulness of the Eating Disorder Inventory with a Non-clinical Population'. *Journal of Counselling Psychology*, 1990, 37, (3), 297–305.
13.   Edwards-Hewitt, T., Gray, J.J., 'The Prevalence of Disordered Eating Attitudes and Behaviours in Black-American and White-American College Women: Ethnic, Regional, Class and Media Differences'. *Eating Disorders Review*, 1993, 1, (1), 41–54.
14.   Gray, J.J., Ford, K., Kelly, L.M., 'The Prevalence of Bulimia

in a Black College Population'. *International Journal of Eating Disorders*, 1987, 6, (6), 733–740.

15.   Garner, D.M., Garfinkel, P.E., 'Socio-cultural Factors in the Development of Anorexia Nervosa'. *Psychological Medicine*, 1980, 10, 647–656.

Chapter 7

1.   Goodman, N., et al, 'Variant Reactions to Physical Disabilities'. *American Sociological Review*, 1963, 28, 429–435.

2.   Kurman, L., 'An Analysis of Messages Concerning Food, Eating Behaviours, and Ideal Body Image on Prime-time American Network Television'. Dissertation abstract, cited by Garner et al in *Anorexia Nervosa: Recent Developments in Research*. New York: Alan R. Liss, 1983.

3.   Bruch, H., *Eating Disorders*. London: Routledge & Kegan Paul, 1974.

4.   Dolan, B., 'Eating Disorders: A Western "Epidemic" Spreads East?' *Eating Disorders Review*, 1993, 1,2, 71–73.

5.   Garner, D.M., Garfinkel, P.E., 'Cultural Expectations of Thinness in Women'. *Psychological Reports*, 1980, 47, 483–491.

6.   Huenemann, R.L, Shapiro, L.R., Hampton, M.C., Mitchell, B.W., 'A Longitudinal Study of Gross Body Composition and Body Conformation and Their Association with Food and Activity in a Teenage Population'. *American Journal of Clinical Nutrition*, 1966, 18, 325–338.

7.   Jakobovits, C., et al, 'Eating Habits and Nutrient Intakes of College Women over a Thirty-year Period'. *Journal of the American Dietetic Association*. 1971, 405–411.

8.   Canning, H., Mayer, J., 'Obesity – Its Possible Effect on College Acceptance'. *New England Journal of Medicine*, 1966, 275, 1172–1174.

9.   Gortmaker, S.L., et al, 'Social and Economic Consequences of Overweight in Adolescence and Young Adulthood'. *New England Journal of Medicine*, 1993, 329, 1008–1012.

10.   Jeffery, R.W., et al, 'Prevalence of Overweight and Weight Loss Behaviour in a Metropolitan Adult Population: The Minnesota Heart Survey Experience'. *American Journal of Public Health*. 1973, 2, 171–177.

11.   Crook, M., *The Body Image Trap*. Vancouver: Self Counsel Press, 1991, p. 6.

12. Metropolitan Life Insurance Company, 'Mortality among Overweight Men and Women'. *Statistical Bulletin*, 1960, 4, Part 1.

13. Clifford, E., 'Body Satisfaction in Adolescence', *Perceptual and Motor Skills*, 1971, 33, 119–125.

14. Orbach, S., *Hunger Strike*. London: Penguin Books, 1993.

Chapter 8

1. Van Praag, H.M., et al, 'Denosologization of Biological Psychiatry or the Specificity of 5HT Disturbances in Psychiatric Disorders'. *Journal of Affective Disorders*, 1987, 13, 1–8.

2. McCargar, L.J., et al, 'Short-term Changes in Energy Intake and Serum Insulin, Neutral Amino-acids, and Urinary Catecholamine Excretion in Women'. *American Journal of Clinical Nutrition*, 1988, 47, 932–941.

3. Hrboticky, N., Leiter, L.A., Anderson, G.H., 'Menstrual Cycle Effects on the Metabolism of Tryptophan Loads'. *American Journal of Clinical Nutrition*, 1989, 50, 46–52.

4. Gladis, M.M., Walsh, B.T., 'Premenstrual Exacerbation of Binge-eating in Bulimia'. *American Journal of Psychiatry*, 1987, 144, 1592–1595.

5. Lacey, J.H., 'Moderation of Bulimia'. *Journal of Psychosomatic Research*, 1984, 28.

6. Hamilton, K., Waller, G., 'Media Influences on Body Size Estimation in Anorexia and Bulimia'. *British Journal of Psychiatry*, 1993, 162, 837–840.

Chapter 9

1. Root, M., Fallon, P., Friedrich, W., *Bulimia: A Systems Approach to Treatment*. New York: Norton & Company, 1986.

2. Pope, H.G., Hudson, J.I., 'Is Childhood Sexual Abuse a Risk Factor for Bulimia Nervosa?' *American Journal of Psychiatry*, 1992, 149, 4, 455–463.

3. Waller, G., Ruddock, A., Pitts, C., 'When is Sexual Abuse Relevant to Bulimic Disorders? The Validity of Clinical Judgments'. *European Eating Disorders Review*, 1993, 1, 3, 143–151.

4. Dolan, B., 'Cross Cultural Issues in the Development, Presentation and Treatment of Eating Disorders', from 'Eating Disorders and Their Treatment' – the proceedings of a symposium held at St George's Hospital Medical School, London, November 1992.

Chapter 10

1. 'Suzanne'. 'All I need for Christmas is a hug'. *Signpost* (the Newsletter for the Eating Disorders Association), December 1993, p. 3.

Chapter 11

1. Lowe, M.G., 'The Role of Anticipated Deprivation in Overeating', *Addictive Behaviours*, 1982, 7, 103–112.

Chapter 12

1. Russell, G.F.M., 'Bulimia Nervosa: An Ominous Variant of Anorexia Nervosa'. *Psychological Medicine*, 1979, 9, 429–448.
2. Hudson, J.I., et al, 'Phenomenological Relationship of Eating Disorders to Major Affective Disorder'. *Psychiatry Research*, 1983, 9, 345–354.
3. Pyle, R.L., Mitchell, J.E., Eckert, E.D., 'Bulimia: A Report of 34 Cases'. *Journal of Clinical Psychiatry*, 1981, 42, 60–64.
4. Hudson, J.I., Pope, H.H., Jonas, J.M., et al, 'Family History Study of Anorexia Nervosa and Bulimia'. *British Journal of Psychiatry*, 1983, 142, 133–138.
5. Piran, N., et al, 'Affective Disturbance in Eating Disorders'. *Journal of Nervous and Mental Disorders*, 1985, 173, 395–400.
6. Levy, A.B., Dixon, K.N., Stern, S.L., 'How are Depression and Bulimia Related?' *American Journal of Psychiatry*, 1989, 146, 162–169.
7. Cooper, P.J., Fairburn, C.G., 'The Depressive Symptoms of Bulimia Nervosa'. *British Journal of Psychiatry*, 1986, 148, 268–274.
8. Tyrer, P., 'Drug Treatment of Psychiatric Patients in General Practice'. *British Medical Journal*, 1978, 2, 1008–1010.

Chapter 13

1. Lask, B., Bryant-Waugh, R., 'Early Onset Anorexia Nervosa and Related Eating Disorders'. *Journal of Child Psychology and Psychiatry*, 1992, 33, (1), 281–300.

2. Bruch, H., *Eating Disorders*. London: Routledge, 1974.

3. Crisp, A.H., 'Epidemiological, Clinical, Diagnostic, Treatment and Prognostic Aspects of Anorexia Nervosa'. In 'Eating Disorders and Their Treatment – Conference Proceedings. St George's Hospital Medical School, London, November 1992.

4. Szmukler, G., et al, 'Anorexia Nervosa: A Psychiatry Case Register Study from Aberdeen'. *Psychological Medicine*, 1986, 16, 49–58.

5. Willi, J., Grossman, S., 'Epidemiology of Anorexia Nervosa in a Defined Region of Switzerland'. *American Journal of Psychiatry*, 1983, 140, 564–567.

6. Fenwick, S., 'On Atrophy of the Stomach and on the Nervous Affections of the Digestive Organs', Churchill, London, 1880.

7. Frisch, R.E., 'Fatness and Fertility', *Scientific American*, March 1988, 88–95.

8. Blinder, B.J., Freeman, D.M.A., Stunkard, A.J., 'Behaviour Therapy of Anorexia Nervosa: Effectiveness of Activity as a Reinforcer of Weight Gain'. *American Journal of Psychiatry*, 1970, 126, 1093–1098.

9. Epling, W.W., Pierce, W.D., Stefan, L., 'A Theory of Activity-based Anorexia'. *International Journal of Eating Disorders*, 1983, 3, (1), 27–46.

10. Crisp, A.H., 'Some Psychobiological Aspects of Adolescent Growth and Their Relevance for the Thin/fat Syndrome (Anorexia Nervosa)'. *International Journal of Obesity*, 1977, 1, 231–238.

11. Garner, D.M., et al, 'Body Image Disturbances in Anorexia Nervosa'. *Psychosomatic Medicine*, 1976, 38, 327–336.

12. Waller, G., 'Why Do We Diagnose Different Types of Eating Disorder? Arguments for a Change in Research and Clinical Practice'. *Eating Disorders Review*, 1993, 1, 2, 74–89.

Chapter 14

1. Carlat, D.J., Camargo, C.A., 'Review of Bulimia Nervosa in Males'. *American Journal of Psychiatry*, 1991, 148, 7, 831–843.
2. Schneider, J.A., Agras, W.S., 'Bulimia in Males: A Matched Comparison with Females'. *International Journal of Eating Disorders*, 1987, 6, 235–242.
3. Salmons, P.H., et al, 'Body Shape Dissatisfaction in Schoolchildren'. *British Journal of Psychiatry*, 1988, 153, 2, 27–31.
4. 'Diet-mad Wives Who Give Their Men a Thin Time'. London: *Daily Express*, 21 July 1993, p. 19.
5. 'The Psychology of Food'. Research carried out by MORI for The Butter Council, London, July 1993.

Chapter 15

1. Redgrave, L., *Diet for Life*. London: Penguin Books, 1993.

Chapter 17

1. Newton, T., Robinson, P., Hartley, P., 'Treatment for Eating Disorders in the United Kingdom. Part II. Experiences of Treatment: A Survey of Members of the Eating Disorders Association'. *Eating Disorders Review*, 1993, 1, 1, 10–21.
2. Robinson, P., 'Treatment for Eating Disorders in the United Kingdom. Part 1. A Survey of Specialist Services'. *Eating Disorders Review*, 1993, 1, 1, 4–9.
3. Fairburn, C.G., in, *The Biology of Feast and Famine*. London: Academic Press Inc., 1992, 317–340.
4. Mitchell, J.E., 'A Review of the Controlled Trials of Psychotherapy in Bulimia Nervosa'. *Journal of Psychosomatic Research*, 1991, 35, 1, 23–31.
5. Coker, S., Vize, C., Wade, T., Cooper, P., 'Patients with Bulimia Nervosa who Fail to Engage in Cognitive Behaviour Therapy'. *International Journal of Eating Disorders*, 1993, 13, 1, 35–40.

Chapter 18

1. Walsh, B.T., 'Fluoxetine Treatment of Bulimia Nervosa'. *Journal of Psychosomatic Research*, 1991, 35, 1, 33–40.

2. Rockwell, W.J.K., Ellinwood, E.H., Trader, D.W., 'Psychotropic Drugs Promoting Weight Gain: Health Risks and Treatment Implications'. *Southern Medical Journal*, 1983, 76, 1407–1412.
3. Fluoxetine Bulimia Nervosa Collaborative Study Group, 'Fluoxetine in the Treatment of Bulimia Nervosa'. *Archives of General Psychiatry*, 1992, 49, 139–147.
4. Report from Drug Safety Research Unit, Southampton England, November 1993, p. 8.

Chapter 20

1. Eating Disorders Association: 'Bulimia: Breaking the Pattern'. Advice leaflet.

Useful Addresses

Many of the following organisations are either run on a voluntary basis or have a very tight budget. When writing to them, please enclose a stamped self-addressed envelope.

Eating Disorders Association
Sackville Place
44 Magdalen Street
Norwich NR3 1JU
Telephone helplines
Over 18 years: 0603 621414 9.00 a.m. to 6.30 p.m., Monday to Friday
Under 18 years: 0603 765050 4 p.m. to 6 p.m., Monday, Tuesday & Wednesday

The EDA has been established as a mutual self-help support organisation which coordinates a network of local groups to help those who suffer alone, those discharged from hospital, and the families of sufferers. It also offers information and understanding through its telephone helplines and newsletters. It does not offer treatment, but does have information about different types of treatment available in each area.

The Maisner Centre
Box 464
Hove
East Sussex BN3 2BN
Telephone: 0273 729818

The Maisner Centre was founded in 1981 by Pauline Maisner who was herself a compulsive eater, and offers help for both men and women with most eating problems. As this is a private service, a fee is charged, but a phone call will give you more information under no obligation.

Diet Breakers
Church Cottage
Barford St Michael
Banbury
Oxon OX15 OUA
Telephone: 0869 37070

Diet Breakers is a national anti-diet organisation working to challenge the 'tyranny of thinness' and helping to break the diet mentality. Most of their work is about self-empowerment and support, and they also offer a ten-week programme, 'You Count, Calories Don't'. Membership is £10 per year, which includes a useful magazine.

Weigh Ahead
2 The Crescent
Busby
Glasgow G76 8HT
Telephone: 041 644 1444

Weigh Ahead was started by Dr Cherie Martin, and is a programme designed to help participants give up dieting, to look at the cause of their overeating, and to learn to eat in response to genuine body hunger.

The Scottish Centre for Eating Disorders
3 Sciennes Road
Edinburgh EH9 1LE
Telephone: 031 667 8642

This centre uses psychotherapy and counselling on a short-term or long-term basis, depending on individual needs. They are also well aware of the importance of self-help and use self-monitoring diaries, raising awareness of triggers which affect mood, etc.

The Princess of Wales' Speech

to the Conference on Eating Disorders, 1993

This is the full text of HRH, The Princess of Wales' speech to the Eating Disorders 1993 conference at Kensington Town Hall, London, on 27 April 1993, and reproduced with her kind permission.

Ladies and Gentlemen, I have it on very good authority that the quest for perfection our society demands can leave the individual gasping for breath at every turn.

This pressure inevitably extends into the way we look. And, of course, many would like to believe that eating disorders are merely an expression of female vanity – not being able to get into a size ten dress and the consequent frustrations.

From the beginning of time the human race has had a deep and powerful relationship with food – if you eat you live, if you don't you die. Eating food has always been about survival, but also about caring for and nurturing the ones we love. However, with the added stresses of modern life, it has now become an expression of how we feel about ourselves and how we want others to feel about us.

Eating disorders, whether it be anorexia or bulimia, show how individuals can turn the nourishment of the body into a painful attack on themselves, and they have at the core a far deeper problem than mere vanity. And, sadly, eating disorders are on the increase at a disturbing rate, affecting a growing number of men and women and a growing number of children, too.

Our knowledge of eating disorders is still in its infancy. But it seems from those I've spoken to that the seeds of this disease may lie in childhood and the self-doubts and uncertainties that accompany adolescence.

From early childhood many have felt they were expected to be perfect but didn't feel they had the right to express their true feelings to those around them – feelings of guilt, of self-revulsion and low personal esteem, creating in them a compulsion to 'dissolve like a disprin' and disappear.

The illness they developed became their shameful friend. By focusing their energies on controlling their bodies, they had found a refuge from having to face the more painful issues at the centre of their lives. A way of coping, albeit destructively and pointlessly, but a way of coping with a situation they were finding unbearable. An expression of how they felt about themselves and the life they were living.

On a recent visit to the Great Ormond Street Hospital for Sick Children I met some young people who were suffering from eating disorders. With the help of some very dedicated staff, they and their parents were bravely learning to face together the deep problems which had been expressed through their disease. With time and patience and a considerable amount of specialist support, many of these people will get well. They and their families will learn to become whole again. Sadly, for others it will be too late.

Yes, people are dying from eating disorders. Yet all of us can help stop the seeds of this disease developing. As parents, teachers, family and friends, we have an obligation to care for our children. To encourage and guide, to nourish and nurture, and to listen with love to their needs in ways which clearly show our children that we value them. They in their turn will then learn how to value themselves.

For those already suffering from eating disorders, how can we reach them earlier before it's too late? Here in Britain organisations such as the Eating Disorders Association are currently being swamped with inquiries and requests for support and advice, so overwhelming is the need for help.

Yet with greater awareness and more information, these people, who are locked into a spiral of secret despair, can be reached before the disease takes over their lives. The longer it is before help reaches them the greater the demand on limited resources and the less likely it is that they will fully recover.

I am certain the ultimate solution lies within the individual. But with the help and patient nurturing given by you the professionals, family and friends, people suffering from eating disorders can find a better way of coping with their lives by learning to deal with their problems directly, in a safe and supportive environment.

Over the next three days, this international conference has the opportunity to explore further the causes of eating disorders and to find new avenues of help for those suffering from this incapacitating disease. I look forward to hearing about your progress and hope you are able to find the most beneficial way of giving back to these people their self-esteem, to show them how to overcome their difficulties and redirect their energies towards a healthier, happier life.

Index

☐	7493 0794 3	**Finding Love, Keeping Love**	Judith Sills £4.9
☐	7493 0526 6	**Coming Back**	Ann Kaiser Sterns £5.9
☐	7493 0936 9	**The Courage to Grieve**	Judith Tatelbaum £5.9
☐	7493 0718 8	**Seeds of Greatness**	Denis Waitley £4.9
☐	7493 1210 6	**Divorce Hangover**	Anne Walther £5.9
☐	7493 1049 9	**Irritable Bowel Syndrome**	Geoff Watts £5.9

All these books are available at your bookshop or newsagent, or can be ordered direct from the publisher. Just tick th titles you want and fill in the form below.

Mandarin Paperbacks, Cash Sales Department, PO Box 11, Falmouth, Cornwall TR10 9EN.

Please send cheque or postal order, no currency, for purchase price quoted and allow the following for postage an packing:

UK including
BFPO
£1.00 for the first book, 50p for the second and 30p for each additional book ordered to maximum charge of £3.00.

Overseas
including Eire
£2 for the first book, £1.00 for the second and 50p for each additional book thereafter.

NAME (Block letters) ....

ADDRESS..

....

☐ I enclose my remittance for ....

☐ I wish to pay by Access/Visa Card Number ☐☐☐☐☐☐☐☐☐☐☐☐☐☐☐☐

Expiry Date ☐☐☐☐

A Full List of Cedar Books

While every effort is made to keep prices low, it is sometimes necessary to increase prices at short notice. Mandarin Paperbacks reserves the right to show new retail prices on covers which may differ from those previously advertised in the text or elsewhere.

The prices shown below were correct at the time of going to press.

JANE R. HIRSCHMANN and
CAROL H. MUNTER

Overcoming Overeating

Conquer your obsession with food

- Lose weight naturally

- Enjoy the food you most desire

- Forget your preoccupation with eating and weight

- Discover the freedom of no restraints

- Give up dieting for ever

Overcoming Overeating makes this all possible, for the authors
have returned eating to its natural place in life, so that food
becomes something to be enjoyed rather than feared.

Concentrating on the normal physiological hunger that we all
experience, Jane R. Hirschmann and Carol H. Munter help you
to break out of the lonely cycle of diet, binge, recrimination and
self-loathing. Both practical and reassuring, they offer radical,
realistic guidance on how to conquer an obsession and restore
the compulsive eater's self-esteem.

'*Overcoming Overeating* will stand out from the crowd of diet
books for its caring response to the compulsive eater.'
  Susie Orbach, author of *Fat is a Feminist Issue*

DR ROY MACGREGOR

The Treatment Handbook

is the equivalent of 300 consultations with your doctor

What might be the problem?

What can you do to treat yourself?

What should you *not* do?

When should you see a doctor?

What should you expect your doctor to do?

How long will the ailment last?

How can you prevent a recurrence?

Thoroughly accessible, practical and informative, this book answers clearly all your questions and worries about symptoms, causes and treatments of a wide range of complaints affecting everyone from babies to the elderly. Compiled by a GP in a busy London Health Centre, and indexed and cross-referenced for easy access, *The Treatment Handbook* is a must for every home.

GEOFF WATTS

Irritable Bowel Syndrome

Until recently, little was known about IBS, a condition
identified by a collection of symptoms which include stomach
pain and discomfort, constipation and/or diarrhoea. For some
people it is no more than a minor inconvenience – for others it
can be painful, and utterly debilitating. Its cause remains largely
mysterious, and no one as yet has come up with a
comprehensive cure. Now this up-to-date, authoritative and
practical handbook covers all aspects of the problem, and
discusses at length its symptoms and treatments. The author
assesses both orthodox and alternative treatments, and gives
invaluable advice about what to do if you are a sufferer.

RACHEL CHARLES

Mind, Body and Immunity

Rachel Charles became fascinated by the workings of the immune system after learning she had cancer. Why had the immune response failed? What could she do to enhance her immune functioning so that she could be permanently restored to health? The answers she found form the basis of this book, which also provides information on other immune-deficient and auto-immune diseases – including allergies, AIDS, rheumatoid arthritis and diabetes – and, using a series of self-scoring quizzes, gives practical advice on how to maintain your immune system in peak condition.

Firstly, listen to any warning signals your body may give you. If you are feeling seriously 'run down', find yourself unable to cope and/or are suffering from chronic anxiety, then don't wait until serious disease strikes. Get professional help now. Then plan your immunity-enhancement programme by making gradual changes in these three main areas: mind and emotions, diet and exercise.

Based on the author's personal experience of fighting cancer and creating a new lifestyle for herself, *Mind, Body & Immunity* draws on the most up-to-date research in the area and provides easy-to-follow, practical guidelines on how you can give yourself the maximum opportunity for good health and long life.

DR CHARLES SHEPHERD

Living with M.E.

It is estimated that there are over 100,000 people suffering from
M.E. in Britain today. M.E. is short for *myalgic
encephalomyelitis*, a term which relates to the parts of the body
affected: *myalgic*, the muscles; *encephalo*, the brain; and
myelitis, the nerves. The principal symptoms are intense muscle
fatigue and brain malfunction following a flu-like infection.

Until recently, many people suffering from M.E. had great
difficulty in finding a diagnosis and a way of dealing effectively
with the disease. This guide provides much-needed basic
information about M.E. The symptoms are described in detail
and there is also information on the viruses thought to be
responsible for M.E., what triggers it and who can get it.
Additional problems, such as disordered sleep, depression, pain
in the joints and difficulties with the eyes, ears and balance are
also discussed.

'A well-researched, up-to-date guide written from an orthodox
medical viewpoint . . . the one to buy for any sufferer who wants
information based on science, not speculation.'
  M.E. Action Campaign Newsletter